CRYSTALS for
KARMIC
HEALING

"Chinese medicine utilizes stones to treat very deep levels of illness—and nothing is deeper than our karmic hindrances. In *Crystals for Karmic Healing*, Nicholas Pearson provides many insightful protocols for cutting through and melting down the stubborn karmic entanglements that prevent us from moving forward in our lives. The information in this book is grounded in his years of experience and contemplation of the minerals and crystals he recommends, and it is motivated by his sincere faith in our potential to heal ourselves, our families, our communities, and our planet."

LESLIE J. FRANKS, AUTHOR OF *STONE MEDICINE: A CHINESE MEDICAL GUIDE TO HEALING WITH GEMS AND MINERALS*

"Nicholas Pearson hits the perfect balance of spiritual knowledge and scientific validation in his book *Crystals for Karmic Healing*. He becomes a personal instructor—sharing his knowledge and standing beside you, guiding you through specific crystals and how they will aid, and sharing step-by-step instructions on crystal layouts for karmic healing. Includes amazing photos and layouts. I highly recommend!"

KRISTI HUGS, AUTHOR OF *CRYSTAL SPEAK* AND *CRYSTAL APPLICATION*

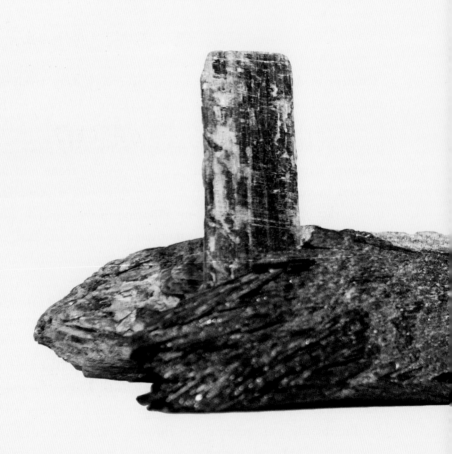

CRYSTALS for KARMIC HEALING

Transform Your Future by Releasing Your Past

NICHOLAS PEARSON

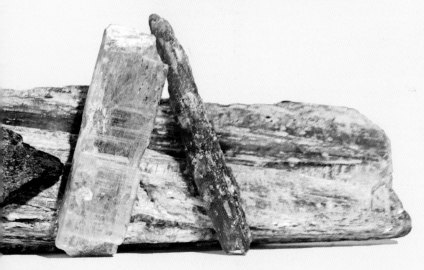

Destiny Books
Rochester, Vermont • Toronto, Canada

Destiny Books
One Park Street
Rochester, Vermont 05767
www.DestinyBooks.com

Destiny Books is a division of Inner Traditions International

Note to the reader: *This book is intended as an informational guide. The remedies, approaches, and techniques described herein are meant to supplement, and not to be a substitute for, professional medical care or treatment. They should not be used to treat a serious ailment without prior consultation with a qualified health care professional.*

Library of Congress Cataloging-in-Publication Data
Names: Pearson, Nicholas, 1986– author.
Title: Crystals for karmic healing : transform your future by releasing your past / Nicholas Pearson.
Description: Rochester, Vermont : Destiny Books, [2017] | Includes bibliographical references and index.
Identifiers: LCCN 2016034335 (print) | LCCN 2016037341 (e-book) | ISBN 9781620556184 (paperback) | ISBN 9781620556191 (e-book)
Subjects: LCSH: Crystals—Therapeutic use. | Karma. | Mind and body. | Healing. | BISAC: BODY, MIND & SPIRIT / Crystals. | BODY, MIND & SPIRIT / Healing / Energy (Chi Kung, Reiki, Polarity). | HEALTH & FITNESS / Alternative Therapies.
Classification: LCC RZ415 .P42 2017 (print) | LCC RZ415 (e-book) | DDC 615.8/52—dc23
LC record available at https://lccn.loc.gov/2016034335

Printed and bound in the United States by Versa Press, Inc.

10 9 8 7 6 5 4 3 2 1

Text design and layout by Virginia Scott Bowman
This book was typeset in Garamond Premier Pro, Gill Sans, Futura, and Stone Sans with Penumbra, Avenir, and Seravek used as display typefaces.
Photographs and illustrations by Steven Thomas Walsh

To send correspondence to the author of this book, mail a first-class letter to the author c/o Inner Traditions • Bear & Company, One Park Street, Rochester, VT 05767, and we will forward the communication.

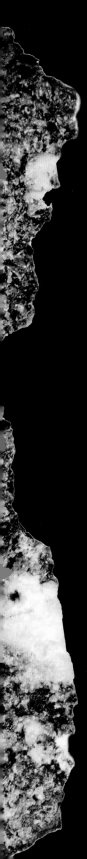

CONTENTS

PART 1
KARMA AND HOW IT WORKS

PART 2

KARMIC STONES AND HOW TO USE THEM

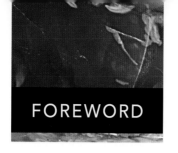

CHANGE THE PAST, RESHAPE THE FUTURE

THIS IS A BOOK I would very much like to have written. Insightful, informative, practical, it brings together my greatest passions: crystals, karmic healing, and astrology—passions that Nicholas clearly shares with me. This book focuses on the karmic release that is so necessary if we are to make the shift into expanded consciousness. We cannot move forward from the Age of Pisces, with its values of money, power, and control, into the longed-for Age of Aquarius, with its values of love, brotherhood, unity, and integrity, unless we clear the karmic and ancestral debris from around us and within us. Now really is the time. Crystals and essences have been two of my core tools for this work, and it's a delight to see that Nicholas has found so many ways in which to use their properties. I'm happy to have contributed to his knowledge, but must add that Nicholas has gone above and beyond what I have published so far by incorporating his mineralogical knowledge in a way that complements his metaphysical understanding. In so doing, he bridges science and spirit—which is exactly as it should be.

If we're on planet Earth at this time, it means we volunteered for the karmic clean-up squad. We all have our part to play. As Nicholas says, the greatest contribution we can make is to clear our own personal karmic patterns, thereby expanding our consciousness. But there is also the question of collective and planetary karma, something for which no one person is responsible, but which nonetheless must be transmuted if humanity is to evolve. We each devise our own way of doing this, and if we have the right spiritual intent, we can then make our tools available so that others can incorporate them into their work if they choose to. It has to be an expanding, cooperative effort if it is to succeed. This book is a giant step on the way to successfully accomplish that goal.

I've been working with crystal grids for many years, so it has been a particular pleasure to experience the grids that Nicholas has devised for karmic clearing. I urge you to try them. Our world needs your contribution!

JUDY HALL

JUDY HALL is an internationally known crystal expert, past-life therapist, karmic counselor, and workshop leader, named one of the hundred most spiritually influential authors by *Watkins Mind Body Spirit* magazine. She has written more than forty books, including the bestselling *The Crystal Bible: A Definitive Guide to Crystals* and *The Book of Why: Understanding Your Soul's Journey*.

ACKNOWLEDGMENTS

MY SINCERE GRATITUDE goes to all those who have supported this project. Thank you to my friend Kat Moyer for helping plant a seed that would eventually grow into the research for this book. To Sharron Britton—many thanks for offering your time, energy, and beautiful minerals for the photography in this book. Thank-you Ariel Albani for the use of your space, and thanks also go to my friends Wakeema, Justin, and Ariel, who stepped in front of the camera to make the exercises in this book come to life. An extra special thank-you is owed to Bob Geisel of Magical Delights (magicaldelights.wordpress.com) for gifting me a Flame of Ishtar stone and sharing his experiences with it. I would also like to extend my thanks to Andy and Sonya of the Princess Sodalite Mine for sending me samples of their exquisite sodalite. Much gratitude to my students, friends, and colleagues who provided feedback during my initial phase of research into this topic. Thank you to the wonderful team at Inner Traditions, especially Jamaica Burns, for helping refine the vision for this book into the text you hold today. Much gratitude flows to Judy Hall for her words of wisdom and kind contribution of her foreword. Most of all, I am grateful to Steven Walsh for his stunning photography and graphics, growing interest and support, and for his overwhelming love and encouragement.

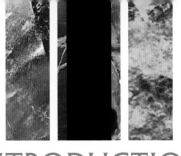

INTRODUCTION

OF THE VARIOUS TYPES of healing available, karmic healing is undoubtedly the most timely and least explored. Karma as a whole is not necessarily good or bad; it is simply the rubric by which your soul's progress is measured. Positive karma, sometimes called *merit*, drives the evolutionary process forward. Unresolved, negative karma is the force responsible for keeping us locked into repeating destructive patterns until we learn the lessons that are being offered by our successive human incarnations.

The time has arrived for karmic healing to take priority among spiritual practitioners. The stage has been set for releasing ties to the past at a rate that humankind has never witnessed. The very universe has prepared us for this turning point in our evolutionary timeline, and the spiritual realms want us to succeed in transmuting the limiting remnants of the past in order to step into the reality of the future. Many people are acutely aware of this shift, and they are leading the way toward new levels of healing.

Karma is accrued on both the personal and planetary levels, while ancestral karma is the karmic pattern inherited from our families and communities. The tools presented in this book can be applied to each and every one of these groups of karmic energies. The higher realms are pointing us toward healing on a much wider scale, and we must accept this task with a sense of urgency. There are myriad tools for assisting this process, and all we have to do is awaken to the moment in order to access them.

The mineral kingdom serves as a unique support system for times of transition; the stones of the Earth have seen more changes than any of us could imagine from the human perspective. Newly discovered rock and mineral formations seem to be deft instruments of evolutionary healing; they have emerged to lend a hand in resolving karmic patterns and accepting our destiny as co-creators of a new reality. We, as a community of healers and spiritually sensitive people, are invited to integrate these crystals into our lives in order to help ourselves and one another. In this way we can wipe the karmic slate clean, or at least clean enough, to initiate a new phase in humanity's development.

USING THIS BOOK

Transforming karmic patterns is not an entirely new premise, yet few texts seem to be devoted to imparting easy and effective techniques for doing so. The first three chapters of this book summarize the main premise of karmic healing by first defining karma and other relevant terms, introducing the spiritual help available for transmuting karma, and creating a context for how to approach karmic healing. This first part focuses on karma as a whole—what it is, how we are affected by it, and how we can now work with it in ways that are unprecedented.

The last two chapters are wholly devoted to how the mineral realm can support our karmic transformation. Rocks and minerals exist outside of the realm of karma, as they generate no negative karma of their own. For this reason they are capable tools for helping to transform karma on a personal or planetary scale. Chapter 4 is an encyclopedic list of the stones and their properties in detail, while chapter 5 describes specific hands-on applications for these tools.

The list of crystals in this work is not final; many other formations will lend themselves to resolving karma in creative ways. Research and experimentation have revealed these stones in my own practice; a similar approach in your own crystal work will unearth more. Wherever possible, I have tried to describe the mechanisms for *why* these crystals work, rather than just discussing *what* they do in a prescriptive manner. Since the subject matter of the book is rather narrow, the stones' effects have only been described within the context of karmic healing; other aspects of their properties have been largely omitted.

Chapter 5 offers a starting point for putting the crystals to work. Many books examine the properties of the mineral kingdom without divulging how to obtain results. In light of this, in *Crystals for Karmic Healing* a diverse array of practices is surveyed, including meditations, crystal grids, gem essences, body layouts, and more. These techniques are like recipes, and you can take your inspiration from them in order to adapt them to your needs. With some experimentation you can integrate the exercises into your own healing practice, either for yourself or for others.

The goal of this book is to inspire you to grow in new ways with the mineral realm. If we as human beings learn to speak the language of stones, we will be able to learn how to adapt to incoming changes and surmount the obstacles that have held us back for lifetimes. The time for moving beyond karmic patterns has arrived, and the stones of our planet are waiting to help us do so.

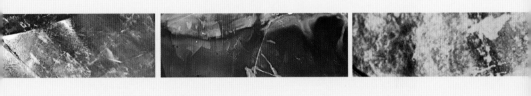

PART 1

✦✦✦

Karma and How It Works

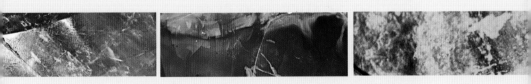

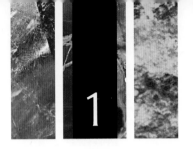

UNDERSTANDING
KARMA

WITHIN THE SPIRITUAL COMMUNITY, *karma* is a buzzword often used to describe the idea of fate or destiny. The term has also been used to imply the pedestrian notion of payback, and for many people that's about as deep as they give karma any thought. In truth, karma is not in and of itself merely relegated to some mystical force of destiny or fate, nor is it a cosmic equalizer that seeks out revenge for misdeeds. Karma is a powerful instrument, a tapestry woven throughout time, over eons, and it represents the sum total of our individual and collective thoughts, deeds, intentions, and actions.

CAUSE AND EFFECT

The origin of the word *karma* can be traced to Sanskrit. Derived from the word *karman,* meaning "action" or "deed," karma is meant to represent the total effect of your soul's progress through many physical incarnations. Although the spiritual concept of karma was first recorded in Hinduism and later in Buddhism and Jainism, it is a concept that permeates many traditions and cultures, as the idea that where you go in this life or the afterlife is predicated on your actions and behavior is not endemic to any one people or culture. The principle of cause and effect is ancient, and it transcends any single population or time frame.

A belief in reincarnation is not mandatory to make sense of karma. Heaven and hell are the results of your choices, actions, and even your thoughts, according to the Abrahamic faiths. Similarly, the ancient Egyptians taught that the heart of the deceased was weighed against a feather in order to determine the fate of a person's soul in the afterlife. Many cultures instead believe in transmigration of the soul, wherein the soul is born again and again through reincarnation and is thus given an opportunity to advance into higher life forms and higher stations in life. Conversely, generating negative karma can result in a similarly backward movement. In this way, the concept of karma is inextricable from the universal law of cause and effect, in which each and every action or choice results in a certain effect or series of effects. This is very much in evidence in the microcosm of our individual lives and is echoed everywhere on a macrocosmic level.

The idea behind karma is the same fundamental principle found in Newton's third law of motion: for every action, there is an equal and opposite reaction. However, karma is not limited to the physical force exerted on material objects. The universe is a dynamic collection of energy fields interacting with one another. Each action or event at the energetic level also exerts an influence on surrounding fields, and this results in an equal and opposite reaction, too. Karma is thus the end result of causal imprints of actions and reactions. In the case of karmic reactions, the energy fields in question and their activities do not necessarily have physical counterparts. This means that spiritual, mental, and emotional energies can incur karmic debts and credits, too.

Karma is the measuring system for our choices in life. We accrue karma from each action and every thought or intention. When our choices limit or harm another energy field, whether it is a person, animal, plant, or idea, we generate a negative karmic imprint, which is a debit in your causal bank account. Conversely, when we engage in choices and behaviors that support and uplift others, we gather good karma—what is known as *merit*—which is a karmic credit to your soul.

This system of credits and debits entangles people at a soul level.

It results in souls that will incarnate together over many lifetimes in order to balance the scales of karma. If your soul has received a gross injustice in a previous embodiment, the enactor of this event will play out the role of equalizing the karma, just as if paying off a monetary debt. Karmic debts inhibit spiritual growth, and they can lead to a variety of challenges in life, including those that affect physical and emotional health.

Causal-level credits and debits are not limited to our own actions and energies. We store information for life at the cellular level, in our DNA. Science has termed many of the sequences in our genes as "junk DNA" because these sequences do not code for protein production or other necessary biological functions. In these seemingly inactive parts of the DNA there is important soul information being stored, such as the spiritual information contained in your soul blueprint. It is here, in the junk DNA, that one finds the energy of karma stored at a subcellular level. This includes the template of our karma from previous lifetimes, as well as the updates we make to our karmic bank account in our current life.

The DNA also holds genealogical karma, which is the karma associated with one's family or tribe. Family constellations therapy, an alternative approach developed in the mid-1990s by German psychotherapist Bert Hellinger, addresses the hidden dynamics of the family into which we are born, including the patterns of mental health, illness, negative emotions, and potentially destructive behaviors that people within families unconsciously adopt. These patterns ultimately are representative of the sum of karmic debits and credits within our families and communities. Genealogical karma offers a unique opportunity to learn lessons associated with the previous experiences of your loved ones and ancestors, as well as predecessors in your communities, organizations, and nations. This level of karma is often very impersonal, and it is more far-reaching than the karma of an individual person. Healing and resolving family-level and group causal patterns has a liberating effect among all members of the target population. Some experiences are so universal that each person incarnated shares in this inherited karma.

On a broader scale, inhabitants of our planet have participated in huge learning opportunities, many of which have contributed to the accumulation of negative karma. Some of these include the fall of Atlantis, wars, famines, slavery, genocides, and many other similar events in Earth history. Even though many people today may have grown past and worked off their own personal karmic debts at the soul level, there is still karmic debris from these planetary events hanging around Earth. And so learning to heal and release karma allows us to not only affect our personal growth in a positive way, but also to contribute to the well-being of humanity as a whole.

Karma is not meant to be viewed as a reward-and-punishment system for our actions. Instead, karma is in place by mutual agreement among all embodied souls in order to facilitate and measure growth. Earth was set up as a learning environment in order to ensure the evolution of our higher selves. It has been suggested by many authors that Creator made humans in order to be able to more fully experience the depth of creation. Because we are individuations from Source (rather than merely *individuals* created by Source), we are representatives of the cosmic, unifying intelligence of the whole. We are here to grow and add to the experience of the soul, thereby propelling the spiritual sparks within us forward toward perfection.

The planet is a manifestation of the choices of its denizens. It emanates beauty, love, healing, and peace, but it also radiates pain, suffering, fear, and entropy. Karma exists in order to resolve the negative aspects of the human condition by facilitating learning at the higher level. Karma helps to imprint the soul's template with information regarding the effects of its actions and thoughts. As these positive and negative patterns accumulate, we experience the effects of our actions through all our lifetimes.

When a particular lesson is painful or difficult, the teaching opportunity is presented again and again. Unlike our current concept of schools, the Earth plane allows you to repeat any exercise or assignment as many times as it takes to fully integrate the lesson. If the same imprudent choices are made more than once, in this lifetime or across several lifetimes, the effects begin to grow exponentially in an effort to help reveal and resolve the underlying lesson. Healing work at the causal, or karmic, level tends to focus on finding the roots of any recurring cycles and releasing or discharging any of the remaining causal information regarding the initial imprint. In doing so, the entire pattern can be slowed, stopped, or erased, depending on the degree of efficacy.

CONCURRENT LIFETIMES

Karma is best appreciated from a point of view that embraces the idea of reincarnation. Rather than a "once-and-done" ideology, reincarnation posits that the soul crystallizes into embodiment over many lifetimes in order to master the lessons of the Earth plane. Several spiritual traditions expand on this idea by teaching that the vessel of the soul is not limited to the human form. This principle, called *transmigration of the soul,* goes hand in hand with the cause-and-effect nature of karmic law. It enables the soul to express growth in many forms and in many lifetimes according to the karmic lessons being learned. These lifetimes include incarnations as plants, insects, and other organisms. In fact, it is possible that some of these lifetimes occur on other planes of existence or on other planets altogether.

In a religious context, the principles of reincarnation and karma are most evident in Eastern traditions, including Taoism, Hinduism, Buddhism, Jainism, and Sikhism. Western schools of thought have also taught reincarnation among their tenets since antiquity. Early Jewish traditions "mention reincarnation quite directly. There are many references to reembodiment in the books of the secret doctrine of the Kabala."[1] Similar views were held by early Christians, including the Gnostic sects, as well as by the Greek Platonists and Socratics.[2] A common principle in each of these reincarnation doctrines is that our decisions in one life have a measurable effect on subsequent incarnations.

The subject of reincarnation has been presented for millennia, and many people experience recall of events from previous lives. Even when no memory or trace of any prior incarnation is evident, the events of the current lifetime are usually shaped by the karma of our former and future lives. Since Earth is a school devoted to soul growth, each incarnation is similar to a new grade level. We are able to repeat a given lesson or grade as many times as is necessary for full integration of the message contained therein.

In reality, although most people describe reincarnation in language that implies linear time, our souls do not experience embodiment with any sense of past or future. Here in the third dimension, time appears to flow forward in a single direction because of our perspective. However, time itself exists at the fourth dimension, outside of the physical universe's measurement of spatial organization. If we lived in the fourth dimension we could move through time just as easily as we navigate the three-dimensional world. The soul is anchored in a much higher plane of reality, and it manifests in all the planes leading up to it. For example, our physical bodies are soul manifestations of the third dimension, whereas our higher selves may be soul manifestations of the fifth dimension. From a higher plane, a new perspective of time is offered. Just as we can survey the entirety of a map, which is a two-dimensional rendering of space, time can be surveyed all at once from the point of view of the fifth dimension. This means that from the higher self's perspective, as well as the soul's perspective, all timelines are simultaneous.

Even if we believe in multiple lifetimes, we tend to assume that we can only influence the current one. Since our true nature is too large to be condensed into a single physical form in linear time, the soul actually crystallizes into many physical bodies in many times, all at once. Using various spiritual tools and techniques such as those described in this book can allow you to explore other lives, irrespective of their time

or location. From the causal perspective, this means that each personality the soul embodies is affecting every other aspect of the soul. In
other words, your karma is the result of every lifetime. Because these
different aspects of the self are happening simultaneously when viewed
from the higher dimensions, it is possible to change the outcome of any
given lifetime, thereby altering or resolving any karmic debts incurred.
To know that you can change or resolve your karma grants you a position of power; instead of being a victim of your circumstances, you can
navigate the causal patterns that have created any challenge in your lifetime. Even if the karmic seeds are leftover patterns from other incarnations, they can be corrected *at their source.* It is actually possible,
through past-life regression and other techniques, to relive or view
past-life events in order to effect change in the current lifetime.

Future incarnations can provide valuable opportunities for healing as well. From the third-dimensional point of view, looking into
forthcoming lives is like peering into a window of your soul's progress. You can actually look to see which lessons you have mastered.
Simultaneously, you can see which challenges are ongoing in an effort
to nip them in the bud in a current scenario.

To experience the healing of karma it is often necessary to trace
the pattern back to previous lifetimes. Engaging in past-life regression
is best handled with a qualified regressionist, although many people
report success on their own. To facilitate the experience of past-life
journeying on your own, various tools can be incorporated into the
process. Helpful guidelines for performing your own past-life regression assisted by the mineral kingdom will be explored in chapter 5.

THE SPIRITUAL BLUEPRINT

Before any part of the universe comes into physical existence, a spiritual counterpart is first formulated in the form of programming
or encoding. This a priori information exists for all levels of existence, from the tiniest subatomic particle to the entire universe. The

information contained represents the idealized state of being for a given creation. Although it is called various names in literature, we will refer to this informational level of premanifest existence as the *spiritual blueprint*.

The blueprint is a manifestation of the causal level of reality, indicating that it exists above and beyond the physical, linear third dimension. Blueprints are constructed as matrices of spiritual information and are primarily composed of color rays (see "Color and Karma" in chapter 3), of which occult philosophy and gemstone therapy agree that there are seven, representing individuated aspects of God or Source.[3]* The color rays are representative of vibrational frequencies or patterns that course throughout the universe; they serve as the fabric from which the spiritual blueprint for any entity, being, cell, or object is formed. The blueprint is a template that serves as the overseeing laws dictating how "the positive, negative, and neutral forces will manifest atoms in the Physical World, [and] they also prescribe how these atoms will interplay with all frequencies."[4] This means that the blueprint is the level of your being encoded for each possible interaction, from the most minute and primordial level on up to the expression of your entire life.

Each time your soul returns to embodiment through the process of reincarnation, a new blueprint is written for that particular lifetime. This blueprint contains a spiritual map of the highest potential that you can express in a given lifetime. Similarly, each cell in your body has its own blueprint, as does each tissue, organ, and organ system. These blueprints are drafted in accordance with your karma; in other words, each lifetime's net karma will directly impact the ensuing blueprint. In this process, karma that is being accrued in your

---

*There are a number of different systems of approaching the seven rays. Throughout *Crystals for Karmic Healing* you'll find references to the color rays, which are the archetypal frequencies of color employed in gemstone therapy. These differ in theory and practice from the seven rays of occult philosophy, especially in terms of their overall simplicity. For more information on the color rays and a brief comparison to the seven rays, consult my book *The Seven Archetypal Stones*.

present lifetime is measured against your blueprint. When karma is not resonating in accordance with your highest expression as defined by your current blueprint, this can be experienced as friction or disharmony in your life.

Each of your past lives has helped to shape the structure and energetic content of your current blueprint. The blueprint itself is the spiritual template responsible for the organizing principles and makeup of each of our physical and nonphysical bodies. These blueprints exist outside of time and space, and they are held within the Akashic records, the compendium of thoughts, events, and emotions believed to be encoded on the astral plane. Personal blueprint information is accessible without having to undergo any form of journeying, as long as the proper catalyst is used, such as the crystal healing tools described in this book.

Your spiritual blueprint exists at the soul level. Because of that, your lower, or earthly, self generally does not have conscious awareness of the information contained in the blueprint. Whenever negative karma is generated, whether from life decisions or from certain mental or emotional patterns, this impinges on your ability to fully express your blueprint's highest potential. In Jainism this is depicted as particles of negative karma that are attracted to you when you, for example, commit a selfish act or even harbor a selfish thought; these particles are believed to dim the light of the soul, just as karma inhibits the expression, or light, of the blueprint. In a healthy person (or cell, or organ, or even a chair), the manifest self is a direct reflection of the blueprint. However, illness, injury, or other challenges in life can result as we drift away from the blueprint's plan.

The good news is that the soul, as well as all the other aspects of any being or object, is able to make a course correction. Typically, the manifest expression, which is the manifest form that the blueprint takes here in the physical world, is able to move into a state of direct communication with the blueprint, much the way that photons can manifest as particles and have a measurable mass, or as waves of energy not composed of tangible matter. This oscillation between states of being happens very quickly so as to be imperceptible to the conscious mind. Each particle of our physical body behaves in a similar way, and it is in this manner that our manifest self can read the information stored in the spiritual blueprint.

It is entirely possible, however, that the process of moving between a manifest and an unmanifest state of being can be slowed down or otherwise impeded by what we do here in the third dimension. Essentially, the karma of each and every thought, intention, word, and action that we choose has the ability to move us into closer alignment with our spiritual blueprint or weigh us down so that we can no longer make adjustments or refinements according to the instructions held by our template. The longer a given aspect of manifestation goes without establishing contact with the blueprint, the more likely it is that illness will manifest.

Merely generating good karma is typically not sufficient for reestablishing contact with one's spiritual blueprint. The state of energetic liquidity, in which manifest reality flows easily between physical form and the premanifest, blueprint state, can be achieved by releasing karmic debris or when catalyzed through the action of specific gemstones.[5] Later on in this book you'll be introduced to a unique group of crystals that may enable healing at the blueprint level.

The spiritual blueprint is also the home of your soul's contracts. These are the agreements your soul made before incarnating that direct your journey on the Earth plane. Your contracts represent your past, present, and upcoming lessons in life. These may take the form of relationships, education, career, spiritual teachings, illnesses, accidents, and many more life experiences. The soul contracts do not imply only limitations or negativity; in many cases the soul writes contracts regarding one's joys and happiness, just as it does one's challenges and obstacles.

When we experience a major lesson in life, especially when it is a difficult one, this is often a premeditated instance in which we lose contact with our soul blueprint and deviate slightly from the idea of manifest perfection. To experience the fullness and richness of our own divine self made flesh, we have elected to grow through both love and pain, through sickness and health. It is often difficult to reconcile the troublesome patches in life; however, your soul recognizes that it is *all part of the plan.* If you are repeating a cycle again and again in life, this is generally a method for your soul to integrate a lesson at the causal, or karmic, level. It is merely an agreement written into your life path.

Because of recent advancements in human consciousness and the overall evolution of our planet, people are now being given an opportunity to rewrite their soul contracts. Many strategies exist for doing so, including the methods described in this book that involve the use of crystals to facilitate this process. Rewriting your soul contract can drastically alter the course of your current incarnation, so the process must be undertaken conscientiously and with a pure heart.

THE AKASHIC RECORDS

The Akashic records are the nonphysical dwelling place of all causal information in the universe. The term *Akashic records* can be traced back to teachings of Theosophy. *Akasha* is taken from a Sanskrit word meaning "sky," "space," or "ether." The records are a vast archive that contains important etheric information related to all aspects of creation. Each thought, emotion, action, and intention from all beings can be viewed in the records. They are traditionally considered to exist on an astral plane, outside of the dimensions of time and space. The events of past lives, future lives, and all events on Earth are available to us in the Akashic records. Each soul contract, karmic pattern, and life purpose is also recorded here. Connecting to the Akashic records is one method for enacting karmic healing, since our karma is mapped out all in one place in these halls.

Finding the Akashic records can be achieved through meditation, astral travel, and connecting with your higher self. The records are available to all, although one must be in the right state of consciousness and have a pure intention for accessing them in order to success-fully do so. Certain crystals also facilitate access to the Akashic records in a variety of ways. Although it is not necessary to visit the records to effect causal healing, each time karma is released or processed, this is chronicled in the Akashic records.

The vast storehouse of information in the Akashic records is an important resource for many intuitive people who access it both con-sciously and unconsciously. Some people are naturally able to view the information contained in the Akashic records, whereas others have the information relayed to them through their higher selves or through benevolent beings who exist at the fifth dimension or higher.

The Akashic records, being outside of space and linear time, are located at or above the fifth dimension. They are soul-level records, and therefore include information on the composition and arrange-ment of each being's spiritual blueprint. Our blueprints are kept in the Akashic records for safekeeping so that they cannot be interfered with by outside influences. Because spiritual blueprints are encoded for the idealized state, they contain instructions for manifesting perfection on all levels of our organization. Blueprints don't generally change just because we cannot express them perfectly, which is why the Akashic records also maintain annals of our karmic patterns or cycles that impede the translation of the blueprint into the physical.

WHY KARMA MATTERS

Karma is much more than just a buzzword among New Agers, as is evi-denced in the aforementioned information. Karma affects your health, abundance, relationships, and growth. We are all programmed to suc-ceed according to the information in our soul's blueprint, but what we do in any given lifetime can either support or suppress our idealized nature. Although it is entirely possible to live a happy, healthy, well-adjusted life without ever contemplating the concept of karma, doing so can give you a leg up on your life's journey.

A glimpse into your karmic patterns can help you understand the "why" behind current events in your life. Recurring themes, repeated relationship mistakes, even chronic health problems may actually have their origins in your karma. Trying to change everything else in life, especially in a way that accrues merit, or good karma, may slowly balance the scales and reverse the cycles of causal debt being paid off. However, returning to the fountainhead of any part of causal reality offers a more effective and long-lasting means of reparation.

The future of your soul's journey is contingent on your karma. Think of your karma as your credit score. An abysmal credit score can prevent an able, driven, and intelligent person from growing in life because of past errors. It takes time to correct through conventional means, and such a person can languish in the meantime. Karma works similarly, for any being who is held back from evolving may soon lose hope and give up on manifesting his or her destiny. Understanding karma can soothe the frustrated emotions of those who are in a "karmic slump." Since much of our karma is generated throughout all of our other concurrent lifetimes, it helps just to know that it isn't something we did in this life, or even in any lifetime in the case of family or group karma. Knowing this typically brings objectivity and peace; there is no need to feel victimized or disempowered. Instead, tremendous change and healing can result from causal healing and karmic release. More importantly, karma matters because we have collectively arrived at a pivotal time in the history of humanity. Massive adjustments in the energies present on Earth at this time are yielding untold shifts of consciousness among all inhabitants of this planet. It is now possible to co-create with the higher planes—an opportunity that has never before been available to us, and as a result we can grow and evolve at an expedited pace.

In light of this, it is critical to know that negative karma that is not cleared or released cannot be permitted into the new, higher-consciousness reality being birthed at this time. For this reason, it is an evolutionary imperative that the karma of our entire planet be amended or erased. The weight of negative karma slows down spiritual unfoldment in the way that carrying a fifty-pound weight inhibits a marathon runner's progress. It is necessary to fix and release the causal patterns of the entire human race in order for the next stage in human evolution to unfold.

We are now being asked to widen the scope of our healing work. As members of society who are the most aware of and passionate about the current shift in consciousness, the spiritual community is tasked with working not only for their individual, personal good, but also for the benefit of all of humankind. Helping others and healing the karma of communities, nations, races, and generations enables humankind to move forward with a clean slate. The evolution of human consciousness depends on the amelioration of karma; without clearing the slate, we are unable to move forward.

Critical mass is defined as the minimum quantity of material, fuel, or energy required to initiate a given reaction. Historically, the critical mass for our next phase of evolution would have required 100 percent of a person's karma to be cleared before any major shift to the higher dimensions. Similarly, the entire planet's sum total karma would have had to have been wiped clean in order to begin the process of planetary ascension or integration. Now, because of the collective spiritual growth and evolution taking place, we are only required to purge 51 percent or more of our karma in order to ascend.[6]* This is a huge gift from the higher realms to humankind, especially since so much has happened to create more and more negative karma down through the ages.

There is more good news. Not only is karmic release so vital in today's world, it is also *easier than ever before.* Unlike previous eras, the generations alive today are being supported by the cosmos and by the higher intelligences who dwell among us on all planes to transmute and

---

*According to the ascended masters teachings, this dispensation was granted by a master known as the Great Divine Director in a channeling, or discourse, given in 1956.

transform our negative karmic patterns. They actively want to witness our success, so they have given us innumerable tools for co-creating at the causal level. Thanks to this singular occurrence by the cosmos and the higher intelligences who dwell among us, we have nearly reached a critical mass. The time to act is now.

THE ROLE OF
THE MINERAL KINGDOM

The mineral kingdom is one of the most significant instruments in our spiritual toolbox. Crystals form as direct geometric expressions of the godhead. As such, the only conscious decision made by any crystal, rock, or mineral is simply to come into form. Any changes or variations from the idealized form expressed in their blueprints are environmental in nature. This means that minerals do not generate their own negative karma. Instead, crystals are meritorious beings who offer up their every available resource for our benefit. The crystal clan is perhaps the most selfless expression of consciousness in physical form. Crystals make their way into every aspect of our lives, from building materials to electronics, from art to science, and everything in between. Minerals are the very substrate on which we live as Earth dwellers.

All crystalline substances are potent catalysts of spiritual change. Crystalline minerals and rocks found in the earth are powerful facilitators of elevated consciousness, miraculous healing, and overall spiritual growth. It is a natural leap to look to the mineral kingdom for help in understanding and releasing karma.

While virtually all stones offer some form of healing, not all are uniquely guided to facilitate karmic resolution. Within the pages of this book you will become acquainted with more than fifty different crystals and gemstones that are excellent tools for causal healing. You will also be given insight into how to apply these tools, which spiritual beings can guide and assist in these processes, and how to direct the focus outward on a global, planetary scale for the benefit of all beings.

Fewer still are those gemstones uniquely attuned to offering healing and integration of the information contained in the spiritual blueprint. However, here again the mineral kingdom offers a unique benefit: because the intrinsic perfection of all crystals is a direct, unrestricted expression of their spiritual templates, being in the presence of crystals begins to encourage a similar relationship with your own blueprint. The more mindfully and conscientiously we spend time with crystalline forms, the more crystalline we become in terms of our spiritual bodies and their inner, holographic perfection.

Crystals are among the first spiritual symbols and tools of the earliest pages in humankind's history book, but they are also leaders in co-creating humanity's future. Everywhere you turn, crystallinity is exploited for its diverse and unending applications in every field. Work with them consciously, reverently, and humbly, and your life will undoubtedly transform.

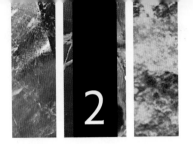

THE LORDS OF KARMA

THE PRIMARY FUNCTION OF KARMA is to track the progress of the soul from one incarnation to another in this school that is planet Earth. With each lifetime, new karma is accumulated, which will either support liberation or require further incarnation. When the soul leaves the body, there is a period of integration of the karmic lessons of the lifetime just passed, which is often referred to as the *life review*. According to different spiritual traditions, the life review may occur in front of a specific audience of angels, Creator, or a group of ascended masters known as the karmic board.

THE KARMIC BOARD

In 1930, Guy W. Ballard, an American mining engineer who was hiking on the side of Mount Shasta in northern California, met the ascended master Saint Germain. As noted by the Saint Germain Foundation, the parent organization of the I AM movement, "Saint Germain revealed many, many things which have been held in secret, and sacredly guarded for many centuries. The Ascended Masters Law of the 'I AM' is the Only Way provided by Life to raise the activity of human beings into the next Octave of Life above the human. It is the Only Way by which individuals can correct the mistakes of the past and go forward free from them in the future."[1] Ballard and his wife, Edna Anne Wheeler Ballard, subsequently founded the I AM movement as something of an offshoot of its predecessor, the Theosophical movement.

In the ascended masters teachings, a group of seven higher-level beings is referred to as the *karmic board*.[2] The members of this group of teachers and ascended masters do not simply pronounce judgment based on the karma that is carried by a soul from any given lifetime. Though their activities span many functions, they are basically tasked "to help man to transmute his evil karma into Divine Light and prepare him to eventually 'return home' via the Ascension."[3] Although the karmic board originally consisted of just three members, they now number seven. Several different compilations of the list of masters serving on the karmic board are available; the list below is derived from the ascended masters teachings and can be found in *The Gnosis and the Law* by Tellis Papastavros. These seven ascended masters are the lords, or in Sanskrit, the *chohans,* of each of the seven rays:

+ **First ray:** Saithrhu
+ **Second ray:** Liberty
+ **Third ray:** Lady Nada
+ **Fourth ray:** Pallas Athene
+ **Fifth ray:** Vista (also called Cyclopea)
+ **Sixth ray:** Kuan Yin
+ **Seventh ray:** Portia

Each of these figures relays the idealized message of his or her ray and helps to integrate the karmic lessons that each ray provides during incarnation.

During the life review, the contents of the causal body are examined. The causal body is a portion of the aura, and it is sometimes referred to as the "memory body" because it contains a karmic imprint of each thought, action, intention, and such contained within it. These form much like the layered appearance of sedimentary rock, and they can be sorted through, band by band. The karmic board is present only to bring causal patterns to the forefront of the soul's awareness; any actual judgment is rendered by the soul itself.[4] Various spiritual texts describe similar interlifetime opportunities to review one's karma. Despite the different names of the gods, angels, or ascended masters who are said to proffer this service, each fulfills a similar task. In this way, the influence of the karmic board and other related spiritual beings may be harnessed in order to take inventory of your lifetime's current karma. Mentally meeting with the board can grant insight into where there are unresolved causal energies or unlearned lessons. With this information, we can make better decisions to redirect our life path toward a healthier, happier route.

It may also be possible to invoke the karmic board to help intercede on your behalf with regard to clearing up any outstanding karmic debts. Since their primary goal is to transmute the karma that weighs the soul down and prohibits stepping into your fully realized, perfected self, the seven members of the board are willing to serve and heal our karmic attachments. Inviting their presence into our life is as simple as mentally asking for their help. Another way to connect to the seven members of the karmic board is through the gemstones that carry the seven rays.

The Ascended Masters and Their Associated Stones

✦ **The first ray of will** is represented by Saithrhu on the karmic board. The gemstone of the first ray is diamond, and other stones connected to this archetypal energy include Herkimer diamonds and other forms of clear quartz.[5] Malachite also supports the right use of will, and it harnesses the qualities of the first ray for resolving karma related to previous misuse of will-power. Topaz taps into the power of will and helps examine the intentions guiding it; in this way it can be used to correct first ray–derived imbalances of intentions that lead to negative karmic patterns.

✦ **The second ray of love and wisdom** is carried by the stone sapphire[6] and is represented on the karmic board by the goddess Liberty. Other second-ray stones include lapis lazuli, sodalite, and azurite. Additionally, rhodochrosite is a stone of freedom, and it can support the work of Liberty.

✦ **The third ray of intelligence** invokes the assistance of Lady Nada; she embodies divine love and is the lord of this ray. Third-ray energy is crystallized in emerald and other Saturnian stones. To invite Nada's mission of divine love into your karmic resolution, try using crystals such as kunzite, pink sapphire, morganite, and lepidolite. Each of these crystals expresses a higher octave of love than mere human love, and in this way they represent Nada's mission. These stones of divine love organize intelligence under the guidance of love itself, which steers karma into the territory of merit.

✦ **The fourth ray of harmony** is represented on the karmic board by Pallas Athene. This ray's primary gem is jasper.[7] Other members of the quartz family, namely chalcedony, agate, and chert, are also conduits for the fourth ray. Pallas Athene's additional role of revealing truth can be brought forth via pietersite, tiger's eye, and turquoise. She is also helpful in revealing how to find a way to live your life's purpose; for this, try using carnelian or citrine to open yourself to achieving your divine mission on Earth.

✦ **The fifth ray of divine intelligence** is represented by Vista. Vista's title is "All-Seeing Eye of God," and he can best be reached through topaz.[8] Other stones that invoke the higher intellect of the fifth ray include golden calcite, yellow sapphire, and fluorite. Lapis lazuli is archetypally related to the all-seeing eye, and it can therefore also be used to invoke the presence of Vista.

✦ **The sixth ray of mercy and compassion** is the territory of the beloved bodhisattva Kuan Yin. Ruby is the crystal of the sixth ray, and its substitutes include rose quartz, pink tourmaline, and most garnets.[9] Additional stones that embody the mercy and compassion of Kuan Yin include jade, pearl, and hemimorphite.

✦ **The seventh ray of ritual, transformation, and magic** is represented on the karmic board by the ascended master Lady Portia. The primary stone of this ray is amethyst,[10] which holds the spiritual energy of the violet flame, too. Tanzanite, charoite, and sugilite may also facilitate a connection to Portia through the seventh ray. Calcite, too, carries Master Portia's energy, for it instills fairness and a fresh perspective necessary to be aligned with the justice that she represents.

CHRIST AS LORD OF KARMA

Architect, philosopher, social reformer, and esotericist Rudolf Steiner (1861–1925), founder of anthroposophy, a philosophical-spiritual movement that centers on human development, posited that "Christ is a cosmic entity who, at a particular moment in history, brought love and the possibility of salvation to humankind by incarnating on Earth."[11] Steiner's teachings were firmly rooted in esoteric Christianity, and his belief was that Jesus, as the Christ, was the redeemer of all karmic patterns. This is evident as one explores the moral ideals taught by Jesus and propagated by mainstream Christianity today.

The predominant moral code of the Western world prior to Christianity was "an eye for an eye," which is an adaptation of the law of cause and effect. Whenever one action is undertaken, a similar event or consequence thusly transpires. Many people have interpreted this expression inasmuch that humans become the instruments for enacting this consequence, despite the fact that the law of karma will see to it that the causal debt is leveled even without human intercession.

However, when the teachings of Christ entered the scene, forgiveness became the law of the people. By "turning the other cheek," we are not surrendering our power or merely awaiting the karmic forces of the universe to exact retribution on our behalf; instead, we are practicing forgiveness and releasing our own attachment to any scenario in which karma can be accrued. In this way we not only help to release the karma of others through forgiveness, but our act of grace also becomes a meritorious deed that accumulates positive karma. In this way connecting to Christ as a spiritual archetype can have a profound effect on our causal patterns, whether we view him as our savior or as an ascended master.

Connecting to Christ in order to resolve negative karma is a practice of forgiveness and surrender. In a surrendered state, there is no attachment to outcome, no grasping, no desiring. In this humbled mode we cannot create further negative karma, because the motivation behind every deed is to be filled with and guided by Christ consciousness. This is the most awakened and refined level of consciousness to which we can aspire; it is the pinnacle of human achievement, the ideal that Jesus represents on the path to enlightenment. Forgiveness furthers this surrendered state, as it releases and absolves preexisting karmic ties. The result is a grace-filled heart and mind.

The only energetic equivalent that can totally eradicate negative karma is grace. We can achieve this beatitude through forgiveness or gratitude, through surrender or self-cultivation. The form itself is less important than the outcome. As we develop spiritual grace, the soul is returned to its pristine innocence, a child-like state of pure potentiality. Now, more than ever, this inspired awareness is necessary. We can make a difference through our relationship with Christ, "who inspires love and forgiveness. Karma continues to operate, constantly bringing balance to our actions. Christ, as Lord of Karma, helps those who trespass to develop a new relationship to their own mistakes and shortcomings, and to others they have harmed."[12]

Stones That Awaken Christ Consciousness

There are a multitude of crystals that may be used to help awaken one's personal Christ consciousness. Chief among them are the Dow crystals, a very special formation of quartz with a precise, mandala-like termination. These crystals express the holographic perfection of the blueprints in all things, especially human consciousness. Because our blueprints are naturally encoded with the potential of perfected realization, they have all the necessary tools for attaining Christ consciousness and thus a release of all karma contained therein. Dow crystals are way-showers, and they point us toward this hidden light within ourselves.

Other crystals and gemstones for awakening Christ consciousness include the diamond, heliodore, golden danburite, selenite, and Herkimer diamonds. High-vibration stones such as moldavite, phenakite, Libyan desert glass, natrolite, scolecite, petalite, and similar stones may have the same effect, as they directly elevate the consciousness. Combining these crystals with any of the karmic healing stones presented in chapter 4 enables you to approach karmic healing through the state of grace, which erases negative karma from the very core of karma's patterning.

SATURN, THE PLANET OF KARMA

According to astrological lore, Saturn has historically been associated with the concept of karma. Named for the Roman god Saturnus, this planet traditionally rules over discipline, structure, order, and time. Saturnus and his Greek counterpart, Cronus, are often depicted holding a sickle or scythe because of their connections to the harvest and its implication of ordered time to bring about the completion of a cycle of growth. Saturn has been given dominion over the passage of time and the realm of karma because of his early association with agrarian calendars and cycles; after all, one reaps only what has been sown.

Saturn's influence is typically viewed as harsh, austere, and restricting. This planet is actually more focused on the underlying infrastructure of any situation than the frills that may distract from understanding. Saturn is disciplined because he understands the

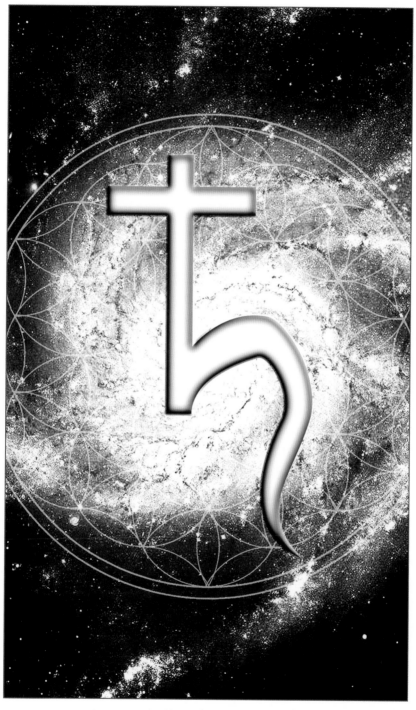

Saturn's symbol

cyclical nature of time and because he prefers substance to fluff in all cases. Saturn, for his early harvest roots, is also a keen advocate of laying the necessary groundwork in order to secure future gains. To be effective, Saturn teaches that you must plan and live according to the natural rhythm of the universe. Imagine trying to plant grain in the winter to harvest in the summer; it just won't work.

As a master of karma, Saturn, both as a planet and as a godform and lord of karma, leads by example. He is a living embodiment of the law of cause and effect. Saturn's message resonates with the principle of form; it is a structural, methodical influence. Because of this, Saturn affects karma by pointing to the patterns that repetitively contribute to our karmic debts and credits. The first step in healing your negative karma is understanding how and why you have accumulated it. For this, Saturn is the most effective teacher.

Beyond revealing the underlying architecture of our karma, Saturn provides awareness of the passage of time. His Greek counterpart, Cronus, shares an etymological root with the words *chronometer* and *synchronize;* he literally guides and guards the passage of time. Anyone under the auspices of Saturn tends to understand timeliness, sometimes all too well. Saturn can offer punctuality, almost to a fault, and it can also open your eyes to bigger cycles in time. Saturn helps to establish right timing in all endeavors, because timing is built on the foundation of understanding the inner structure of a given concept.

In causal healing, Saturn is the reaper of effects as equally as he is the sower of seeds. The influence of Saturn can be invoked when you need better clarity in your karmic healing. Because he can be restricting and limiting due to his austerity and coldness, the planet of karma can help congeal or slow the passing of events in order to grant a better perspective on how things will play out. Saturn also improves our ability to plan with regard to patterns, cycles, and rhythms, especially from a wider point of view than we usually take. Saturn's energy can offer an idea of where we are in the sequence of events that is unfolding, which means that we can make adjustments according to our expected trajectory.

Saturn does not necessarily offer healing or release of karma; rather, he tends to exact karmic justice by ensuring that cycles align as they are supposed to. However, because Saturn expands our vista, we can make a course correction by acting on the limitations that the planet reveals. Saturnian energy is also often employed for banishing unwanted influences from our life, which can sometimes be translated to causal energy. Saturn helps to rid our life of the unwanted so that we can redefine the structure around which our life path is organized.

Saturn and Associated Stones

There are several ways to access Saturn's archetypal effects in working with crystals. In alchemical lore, lead has been aligned with the properties of Saturn, and so lead-bearing minerals provide a direct link to the planet's influence. These include galena, cerussite, vanadinite, crocoite, pyromorphite, mimetite, and wulfenite, among many others. Similar to how Saturn is related to the skeletal system, lead ores reflect the same patterns and bonds that calcium offers. Pyromorphite especially resembles the structure and composition of apatite, which is an integral component in our bones. Use lead minerals to bring a form-minded approach to karmic resolution, as well as to emphasize the course of causal energy. They help identify the skeletal components supporting and linking karmic events. In chapter 4 you'll find detailed descriptions of galena and cerussite, both ores of lead, and amazonite, which contains trace amounts of lead.

Other ways to connect with Saturn's energy include indigo ray stones, as modern Western occult teachings connect Saturn to the color indigo. In gemstone therapy, the indigo ray is ascribed to the influence of form and structure, including the skeletal system, all of which are the traditional domain of Saturn. Traditional magical and ritual correspondences also link indigo to Saturn, as indigo is the color ascribed to Saturday, the day of the week ruled by and named after Saturn.

The indigo ray stones, especially crystalline indigo-colored sodalite, described in chapter 4, also emphasize structure and form. With an understanding of the underlying structure of past events, they allow you to better estimate future outcomes. As this becomes more refined, your intuition actually significantly increases, which enables you to see how karma will continue to influence you.

Some traditions also associate the third ray, represented by the color green, with the rulership of Saturn.[13] In these instances, harnessing the power of such stones as emerald, malachite, aventurine, and imperial jade can also provide some of Saturn's insight. Vedic astrology uses blue sapphire to engage the positive traits of Saturn, including patience, spirituality, organization, and a good moral compass.

OTHER GODS AND GODDESSES, GUIDES, AND MASTERS

Building a relationship with other members of the spiritual hierarchy may assist you on your path to karmic resolution. It may take some time to experiment with the archetypal thought forms and energies composing these beings so you can find a good vibrational match. Because it is vital to build a personal connection to these energies, more options include the following:

✦ **Archangel Zadkiel and Ascended Master Saint Germain** are associated with the seventh ray. They are masters of transmutation and help to bestow the freedom of karmic grace through spiritual alchemy. The primary tool for achieving this is the violet flame, which will be discussed in greater detail in chapter 3.

✦ **Omri-Tas** is a galactic-level ascended master associated with the violet flame. In the ascended masters teachings, Omri-Tas is the ruler of the Violet Planet, a celestial body that exists on the etheric plane very far from Earth. His planet is responsible for transmitting the violet flame to our own world; he is therefore a helpful guide in requesting the power of the violet flame to transmute one's karma. All of the guides and masters connected to the violet ray can be accessed through amethyst (see chapter 4). Other violet-ray stones include charoite, purpurite, lavender quartz, purple fluorite, and purple tourmaline.

✦ **Serapis Bey** is the lord, or chohan, of the fourth ray, and he plays a vital role in the ascension process. His goal is to raise the consciousness of humankind until it is aligned with awareness of the immanent divinity. His teachings focus on healing through grace, and he grants liberation on the causal level through karmic grace. Clear calcite, a detoxifying stone, instills the connection to Serapis Bey.[14]

✦ **The Fates,** also called the Moirai, are a group of goddesses who are said to weave the fabric of time and destiny. Though the concept is Greek, they have analogs in many cultures around the world, including the Norns and the Wyrd Sisters. Although we are gifted with the free will necessary to rewrite our destiny, these goddesses can be invoked to amend the agreements we have made before birth, the soul contracts. Connect to them through obsidian (see chapter 4), which takes you into the cosmic void out of which their tapestry of life is woven. Moonstone, especially dark gray and black varieties, can help to reveal what is hidden, such as the clauses in our soul contracts, and it will help connect to the Fates' knowledge of your destiny. Because they are linked to the ideas of time and fate, fossils also unite us with the Moirai, especially petrified wood (see chapter 4).

✦ **Archangel Michael** is another excellent facilitator of karmic healing. His mission is to release our fears and protect us from temptation, which presents the accumulation of negative karma. The mighty sword that he carries may be invoked to cut through the illusion of the third dimension as well as any karmic ties that we experience through incarnating in the third dimensional realm. He is especially helpful during the karmic cord-cutting exercise described in chapter 5. Blade-like crystals such as selenite (see chapter 4) and various types of laser wands are symbolically in tune with Michael because of his sacred weapon. Other crystals that invoke his influence include amethyst (chapter 4), fire agate, flint (chapter 4), fire opal, hematite, and labradorite.

✦ **Raziel** is an archangel whose name means "Secrets of God."[15] One of his many talents is in interpreting past-life memories, and he can guide us in the dreamtime in order to reveal the imprints of our concurrent lifetimes. Call on his help with diamond (chapter 4), agate, apophyllite (chapter 4), azurite, obsidian (chapter 4), and topaz.

THE IMPORTANCE OF REQUESTING HELP

Merely knowing which aspect of the divine rules over karma is unfortunately not sufficient for getting an ascended master involved in one's causal healing. There is an entire spiritual hierarchy of angels, ascended masters, guides, our higher selves, and Source (in all its many forms) just waiting to step in and help get our lives in order. The key is that they cannot do so without our *express and direct permission*. The beauty in this is that the entire heavenly host is only an invitation away. By consciously asking for their assistance, these spiritual beings are able to intercede in our lives. They offer healing and help physically, mentally, emotionally, spiritually, and karmically. Virtually every emanation of Source is willing to gently guide and correct your course.

To take advantage of these higher intelligences and their miraculous interventions, you can spend a moment in silent prayer or you can create an elaborate ritual; whichever style matches your spiritual practice will provide the outcome you seek. In the case of working with gemstones, any crystal can be imbued with a specific intention, such as summoning the cooperation of the heavenly realms. Selecting an appropriate crystal is the first step; follow up with acknowledging your intention. If Saint Germain's alchemy is your desired tool, start with an amethyst and ask for the help of beloved Saint Germain. You can then program the stone according to the instructions in chapter 5, specifying that it will be a tool to connect you with the transmutative gifts of Saint Germain. Similarly, any other stone can be aligned with the appropriate being or guide.

Resolving lifetimes' worth of karma is not an overnight gig; it requires diligence and discipline in order to obtain the desired outcome. When we ask for divine intervention, we are gifted with an augmented capacity to restore karmic balance to our soul, thereby freeing it to better express its innate perfection. Clearing out the causal debris lying between your current state and the idealized state prepares us for evolution. As mentioned in chapter 1, we have nearly reached the critical mass needed to shift the planet into higher consciousness. The spiritual realms want to see humanity succeed in our mission to master the lessons of Earth school. To take the next step forward, releasing and transmuting our karma is imperative; we cannot grow any further without clearing the causal impediments we have created. Call on the guides, gods, angels, and masters with whom you resonate in order to accept the myriad blessings that are available now.

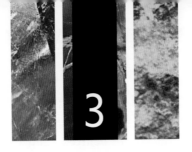

WORKING WITH KARMA

TO BETTER UNDERSTAND how crystals can help us resolve karma, it is first necessary to gain a clear comprehension of how to access causal patterns and karma. Causal patterning is mostly stored in specific aspects of the subtle anatomy, including the aura and chakras. Knowing where to find this karmic energy is half the battle in healing it; once these target zones are located, the karmic healing stones in chapter 4 can be applied for resolution of the causal patterns trapped there. This chapter will describe where to find the stored memory of karmic patterns, how color is helpful in resolving karma, and several other methods for initiating karmic healing.

WHERE KARMA LIVES

Causal information is held in the aura in the causal body, also referred to as the causal aura, karmic body, or the ketheric template.[1] The aura as a whole is a torus-shaped field of energy radiating outward from our body. It is measurable by conventional science and is composed of various parts of the electromagnetic spectrum. Additionally, the aura contains spiritual energies and imprints not yet identified by science that are organized into different bands or layers. Because many different paradigms exist for diagramming the layers of the aura, the causal body is sometimes depicted as the seventh and outermost layer of the aura, whereas other sources place it as the third major layer around the

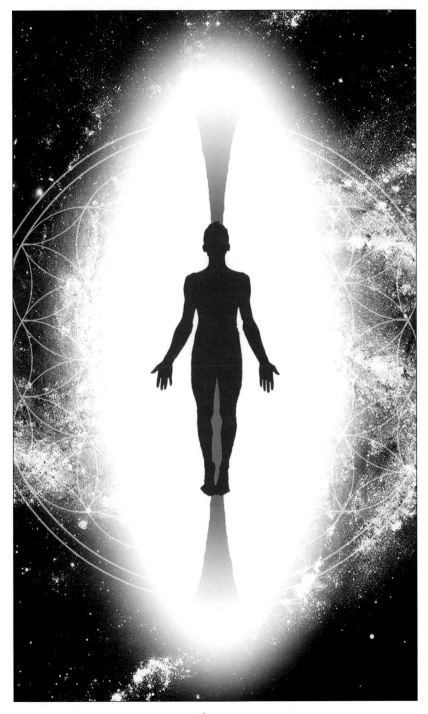

The aura

physical body. Generally, authorities agree that this band of the aura is approximately two to three feet away from the body in an average, healthy aura.

According to Theosophical teachings, the causal body is formed when the soul is first extended from Source.[2] As the newborn spark of the soul, or I AM presence, leaves the heart of Creator, it passes through seven spheres of influence corresponding to the seven rays. These concentric circles are not unlike an aura, with its seven major subdivisions encircling the godhead. As the soul journeys through each of the seven spheres, the causal body is built up and imprinted with each of the colors in the spectrum.

It is necessary for a soul spark to exhibit and integrate all seven archetypal frequencies in the causal body before it is able to begin incarnating into a physical vehicle. The seven rays represent the cosmic principles and patterns out of which our blueprint is formed, and without a particular frequency we are incomplete beings. Any sphere in which we spend more time than the others as newborn souls leaves a wider imprint in the causal body. This explains why we each have different causal backgrounds, strengths, opportunities, and lessons to learn.

The causal body is also considered the "memory body" of the aura because it maintains a record of all the events witnessed and experienced by your consciousness. Its primary function is to store, sort, and stabilize karmic patterns. A healthy causal body can resolve and release karma with relative ease, allowing the necessary credits and debits of causal energy to flow without inhibition. Even when karma is altered or transmuted, this is recorded in the causal body, a process used during the life review between incarnations.

The composition of this level of the aura displays pronounced bands, like the strata in sedimentary rock. These represent memories, karma, and past lives. In a typical aura, as past-life information and karmic cycles are awakened or triggered, the information stored in the causal body springs into action. When mental, emotional, or other

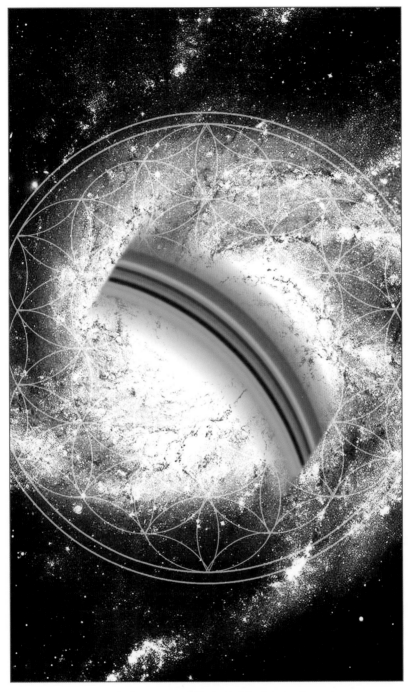

*The structure of the causal body reveals
sediment-like bands of memory.*

aspects stimulate the causal body, ties or connections between corresponding levels of the aura and chakras will occur.

These interenergy connections should be temporary, and they serve as lines of communication while karmic energy is interpreted and processed. In an unhealthy aura, causal energy can get stuck in this formation, thus inhibiting the proper release of karma. In these cases it is necessary to disentangle the causal information from the other bodies or chakras before it can be sufficiently resolved or released.

Since the causal body acts as a repository of memories, each time we incur new karma, either positive or negative, it is recorded in the karmic body. Virtually every emotional, mental, and physical experience, whether it is traumatic or comforting, will be stored here. Even when a particular opportunity for healing such as a painful emotional experience or mental dysfunction is remedied, a counterpart will remain in the memory body. This means that even when we release and recover emotionally, mentally, or physically, we must also address the causal body in order to prevent symptoms or cycles from recurring.

To access the causal body during the application of crystals and gemstones, a topic discussed in greater detail in chapter 5, the stones may be moved or swept through the aura at approximately the height of the causal body (two to three feet away from the body or greater), or they may be placed at certain target points, like at the causal chakra, described below. Golden beryl, also called heliodor, is the most nourishing gemstone for the causal body.[3] Golden calcite, banded opal, and selenite are also beneficial.

ADVANCED CHAKRAS FOR CAUSAL HEALING

Understanding the chakras offers another window into comprehending the human energy field and how it works. Derived from the Sanskrit word for "wheel," a chakra is a vortex of energy that is part

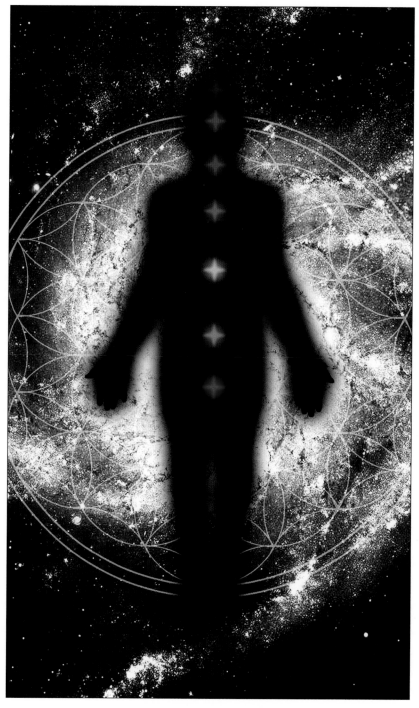

The seven major chakras

of the nonphysical anatomy. These funnel-like, helical formations are mostly situated at major nerve ganglia, glands, other organs, or along other major anatomical features of the body. The chakras act as windows through which spiritual information is relayed to the physical anatomy. Healthy chakras are symmetrically shaped and, in most cases, extend both forward and backward from the body into all layers of the aura.

Most literature focused on healing describes seven major chakras and their domains, while ancient texts on the subject of spiritual anatomy depict hundreds, sometimes thousands, of other, minor energy centers throughout the body. While a seven-chakra system has been sufficient for the last epoch in human evolution, new information suggests that as we receive new energies to support the planet's transformation, our spiritual anatomy has begun to evolve toward a new paradigm. Many modern spiritual teachers have begun to focus on a twelve-chakra system as a response to the evolutionary processes now unfolding. While the exact placement of these chakras may differ based on the source, the basic premise seems universal. Several of the formerly minor chakras have begun to step up to the role of becoming major energy centers in the body.

Of these formerly minor chakras, the earth star and soul star chakras are probably the most important. Considered transpersonal chakras, they actually exist outside the confines of our physical body, nestled within the openings in the bottom and top of the toroidal field of energy encapsulating the physical body that is the human aura. The earth star and soul star are gateways on each end of the aura to ensure a healthy exchange of energy between the planet and the higher realms. The soul star chakra is located approximately six inches above the crown chakra, where it serves to heighten one's relationship to the universe, allowing the soul to ascend beyond the human ego. The earth star chakra is located approximately twelve to eighteen inches below the souls of the feet, where it connects the body and the soul to the powerful energies within the magnetic core of planet Earth; the earth

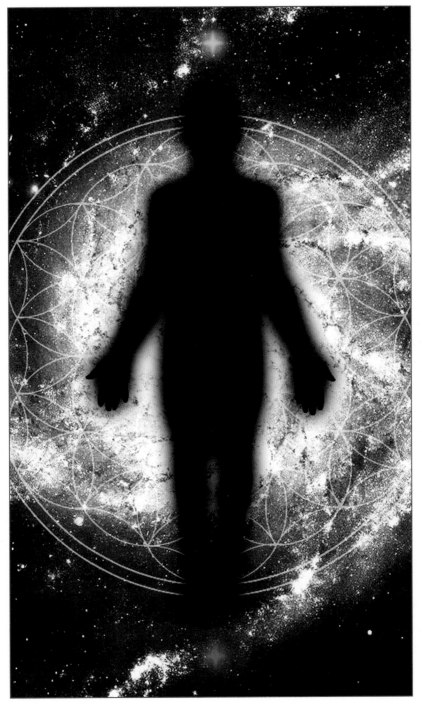

The soul star and earth star chakras

star chakra holds the keys to past lives, karmic patterns, and DNA origins.

While several colors work with each center, white or gold is the most nourishing to the soul star, and black and metallic colors vitalize the earth star. The soul star chakra is best activated with selenite, and golden beryl is also effective. Diamond, danburite, and phenakite are also applicable. The earth star is stabilized and nourished with hematite, and it can also be supported by cuprite, black tourmaline, shungite, and black or carbonado diamonds.

Another of the advanced or emerging chakras is the causal chakra. This energy center is located on the surface of the head approximately four inches behind and slightly below the crown chakra; it helps to align and integrate the energy coming into the field through the soul star chakra. Its function is to bring peace and initiate a higher level of mental awareness of the spiritual self. The causal chakra provides an understanding of how our minds shape our reality. It can yield comprehension of the blueprint and the underlying form of karmic patterns. The causal level is the most rarefied aspect of all the bodies in which our minds operate. It is at this level that the law of cause and effect works most clearly to transubstantiate the light patterns of the divine mind into physical reality. Although it is at the far stretches of the mind, the causal plane acts as a stepping-stone between the highest dimensions and physical reality.

When fully activated, the causal chakra assists perception and works as a filter for the conscious mind in order to streamline the mental energies with their corresponding causal blueprint.[4] This can reduce the action of the ego on our thoughts and offers deep spiritual inspiration. When integrated into our practice, the causal chakra enables higher learning in order to establish your divine presence on Earth, thereby facilitating the unfolding of your destiny and the generation of positive karma, or merit. The causal chakra works closely with the layer of the aura called the causal body in processing karmic patterns. Karmic patterns are sorted and assimilated through the

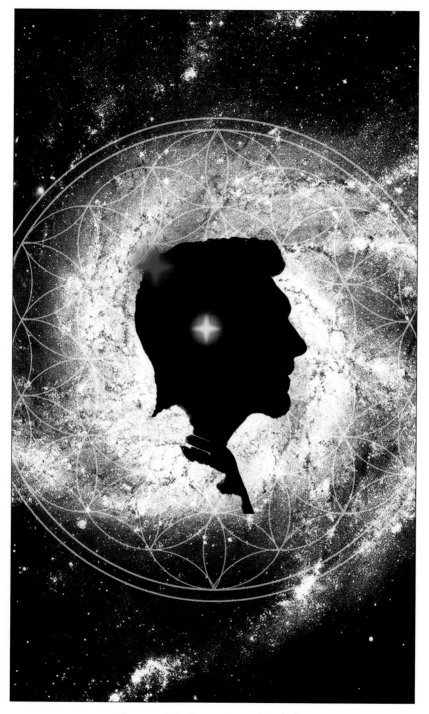

The causal chakra and past-life chakras

cause-and-effect perspective of the causal chakra before being stored in the causal body.

The causal chakra is activated by kyanite.[5] It is sometimes associated with the colors magenta and indigo. Other crystals associated with the causal chakra are amethyst, selenite, labradorite, and celestite.[6]

The past-life chakras are twin chakras located on each side of the skull, at the bony ridge just behind the ears. These minor chakras hold memories of the past, and they receive, process, and store information from concurrent lifetimes. By massaging them or stimulating these minor chakras with crystals, memories can be recalled. These usually occur as brief glimmers or scenes from past lives. The past-life chakras are subtle portals to listening to the echoes of our ancestors, and they may be used to remediate family karma, especially when the second chakra, which governs all of our relationships, is accessed in tandem.

Crystals such as amber, fossils, amazonite, gabbro (especially the variety known as blizzard stone), dumortierite, flint, and wind fossil agate are among the most efficient tools for working with the past-life chakras. Many of the other crystals described in chapter 4 may also be used with success. Opening and clearing these centers facilitates memory, past-life awareness, and clairaudience. Wearing earrings of any of the relevant minerals is a simple way to offer gemstone support to these energy centers.

Additionally, each of the seven major chakras communicates with the causal body, just as they do with each of the other layers of the aura. Therefore, you can work with any chakra whose influence includes the particular lesson presented through causal patterning. Please consult an appropriate resource if additional information on the chakras, both traditional and emerging, is needed in order to facilitate karmic release.

COLOR AND KARMA

The world around us is made more detailed and enriching through the experience of color. Color has a profound effect on the mind, even to the extent that it can change brain chemistry, signaling a domino-like sequence of events in the body. It has an ability to create tangible, achievable results in a number of ways.

Colors are only a small part of how crystals work. Crystal healer, educator, and author Naisha Ahsian teaches that the color of a gemstone represents only about one-sixteenth of its total sum of energy, so clearly it is limiting to group crystals solely by their appearance. With that in mind, however, consider how paint color is chosen to affect the inhabitants of certain rooms, and why advertisers select colors that encourage consumers to spend money.

Color therapy with gemstones is usually focused on matching up a colored gem with an appropriate chakra. Although this model works for many, it assumes that the color of a gem is its defining factor, rather than its composition or morphology. As important as color is, many factors contribute to the total effect a mineral has on one's well-being. Bearing that in mind, gemstone colors can be an excellent starting point for many practitioners.

In addition, certain gems have a unique property of serving as the anchors for each of the seven color rays on the planet that are representative of certain vibrational frequencies found throughout the universe (discussed in chapter 1). In this way, the color ray–bearing gemstones can have profound effects in healing.* Although an in-depth study of the seven color rays is beyond the scope of this book, understanding how to apply color and colored gemstones to

*In gemstone therapy, the color rays are each anchored to our planet by specific gemstones. The color ray gems are ruby (red ray), carnelian (orange ray), yellow sapphire and citrine (yellow ray), emerald (green ray), blue sapphire (blue ray), indigo sodalite (indigo ray), and amethyst and purple tourmaline (violet/purple ray). They are described in detail in *Gemstone Energy Medicine* by Michael Katz (pages 40–42).

the resolution of karma is a subject worthy of exploration. Below are brief descriptions of various colors and their effects on the causal body, karmic patterns, and other aspects of our lives that are affected by karma.

✦ **Black** facilitates journeying into the unknown. It represents the void of becoming and the shadows we lock within ourselves. Black crystals can be good purifying stones, as black pigments absorb all wavelengths of light in the visible spectrum. Black can also represent the power to push through blockages and fears.

✦ **Blue** is a mental color, and it helps ease discomfort of the mind. In karmic healing it strengthens the mind in order to identify, understand, and relate causal information. Many blue stones relate to dialog, whether through physical communication, such as amazonite, or through the interplay of energy, such as kyanite. Blue can offer a freshness that supplants stale and stagnant energies, and it can conversely help to instill calm amidst turbulence.

✦ **Gold** is especially nourishing to the causal body. Golden, translucent crystals such as heliodor or calcite can strengthen and uplift the causal layer of the aura, thereby making it easier for other stones to sort and sweep away patterns of karma from within it. Gold is also representative of joy, wealth, and vitality, and it can help to emphasize the right use of the will. Apply golden energy in order to link the crown and solar plexus, as well as to help break free from situations that disempower you.

✦ **Green** is strongly healing and nurturing. It indicates new growth and health, as well as bringing to mind physicality. Green is traditionally the color associated with the third ray, and therefore also the planet Saturn. Green helps to counteract the inertia of karma by inviting new movement and ideas to develop. Green also reminds us that the physical body is a vehicle for spirit and that the physical world is a classroom for the soul. From this perspective, karma can be looked at objectively, or even with gratitude, as a tool for learning. Green may also be used for healing your relationship with money and the karmic roots of any negative patterns therein.

✦ **Indigo** conveys the Saturnian influence of structure and form. Indigo is the color ascribed to the third eye in modern literature, and it confers intuition and insight, as well as a steadfast and resolute commitment to what is below the surface of any event or idea. Indigo has a contemplative nature, and this helps provide a glimpse into causality and the law of cause and effect.

✦ Orange overflows with charisma, vitality, and energy. Crystals that form as expressions of this color tend to exert an uplifting influence over those who wear and hold them. Orange sets us up for success by boosting confidence and belief that hard work is all it takes. Orange minerals can help one to push through limitations and karmic patterns through a necessary boost of energy. Orange may be applied to heal the karmic underpinnings of sexual hang-ups and obstacles.

✦ Peach blends pink and orange, and it bridges the gap between the emotional and the causal energies in our aura. Peach gemstones can help to soften raw emotions built around any karmic tie or cycle. Use them to extricate karmic patterns from the emotional body, thereby encouraging you to set them free altogether.

✦ Pink speaks to the heart; it gently feeds the emotional body and the heart chakra. When strengthened, our emotional aspects of self can move forward in overcoming difficult karmic lessons. Pink stones may also be useful in softening the effects of karmic release and in understanding the causal relationships we experience interpersonally. Combining emotional healing stones with karmic healing stones can effect profound changes in our relationships.

✦ **Red** burns through blockages, especially in our physical and emotional bodies. Less suited to karmic healing than other colors, it still offers aid to finding passion and using survival skills to undermine negative karmic patterns. Red may offer much-needed grounding and strength, and it can stimulate forward momentum during karmic release in order to break free from the staid inertia of causal cycles.

✦ **Violet** (or purple) is the most profound frequency for karmic transmutation. It brings spiritual awareness to any karmic pattern, and it helps you to be of service to humankind through your spiritual work. Use violet to connect to the seventh ray and the violet flame for spiritual alchemy on a personal and planetary scale. Purple energy seeks out limitations in order to release their hold over us, and this action can be effectively and simply applied to karmic healing through the use of the violet flame.

✧ **White** and colorless gemstones often connote a purity of spirit. White is an amalgam of all the wavelengths of visible light, and it helps to achieve balance and perfection. Some of the most important stones for karmic transformation are in this category, including quartz, diamond, and apophyllite, and they are potent activators of spiritual development. White and clear stones can help to clear the karmic debris limiting the expression of our blueprints.

✦ **Yellow** inspires creativity and flow. In karmic resolution it can help in the processing and elimination of karma by vitalizing the mechanisms that help discard and release old cycles. Yellow works closely with gold, and each can support the other. Many yellow gemstones also invite the right use of willpower to align our personal power to the higher power.

KARMA AND THE DREAMTIME

Each and every day is replete with scenarios in which you are able to add to or change your karma. Every decision you make either benefits you and others with a credit of good karma, or slows down your progress with negative karma. Since this is a continuously unfolding process, your mind and your higher self need an opportunity to review and process this stream of causal information on a daily basis. This is accomplished during the dreaming state, when the causal body is the most active.

Dreams are doorways to other planes of consciousness, and they serve a multitude of functions. Some dreams may be spiritual journeys, meant to invite growth or healing. Others can be manifestations of the intuitive mind, wherein they relay important information regarding one's future. Most dreams, however, fall into the category of a review of events. Sometimes these events are from the recent past, while other dreams may dredge up memories from the most distant reaches of the mind.

The causal body serves as the aura's memory drive. It contains a record of every thought, feeling, intention, and action we have undertaken, in this life and beyond. Because this amount of information is much too great for the conscious mind to handle, the causal energies are best sifted through during sleep. Dreaming unlocks portions of the mind that may otherwise not be used while simultaneously circumventing the influence of the ego and the conscious mind altogether.

Dreamtime is a term that refers to a level of nonordinary reality, a shamanic or astral plane of existence. It is derived from a concept found in the aboriginal culture of Australia, and it refers to a place that exists outside of time. It is eternal, uncreated, and nonphysical. In this realm the ancestors dwell, as do other spiritual beings who can offer their teachings to humanity. The dreamtime is the place our spirits journey to during sleep and other altered states of reality in order to process causal information for the benefit of the soul's continued education.

Dreamtime journeys involving causal information help the entire being sort out ongoing karma. This is why a memory from the distant past can be accessed in the dream state even when we do not think about these events during waking consciousness. Oftentimes, these memories have strong emotions attached to them, and our dreams can seemingly open old wounds. The truth is that the karma from these events is still relevant to our daily lives, and our dreams enable us to work through and integrate karmic lessons in order to move beyond the limits they present.

Since our dreams are geared toward resolving karma, it is possible to make a conscious effort to enhance their efficacy. Setting an intention or reciting an affirmation before falling asleep can help align all the aspects of your being with a common goal, such as karmic healing. You can also sleep with specific crystals or gemstones that support this work. Many karmic healers are also wonderful crystals for improving the quality of sleep or enhancing the vividness of dreams.

Opals in matrix, like boulder opal and banded opal, are wonderful dream stones. They support the work of the causal body, and the side effect is that they will relax the conscious mind into deeper sleep in order to facilitate the causal body's functions. Similarly, chrysotile, heliodor, and kyanite can improve sleep.

Certain crystals focused on astral travel and past-life journeying are also helpful during the dream state. Try using apophyllite, flint, and petrified wood during your slumber in order to facilitate more effective journeys and more vivid dreams. Phantom crystals, record keepers, trigonic crystals, and time link crystals are also sacred stones with a huge impact on your dreamtime adventures. For best results, cleanse and program your crystals prior to placing them beneath your pillow. Instructions on how to cleanse and program crystals are included in chapter 5.

PAST-LIFE JOURNEYS

One way to address the origins of a karmic pattern is through reliving the lessons of concurrent lifetimes. A myriad of systems exists for doing so, many of which are hypnotic regressions facilitated by a qualified therapist. Although having a practiced guide enables a clearer, easier regression, it is possible to journey into past lives on your own through meditation. Various types of imagery are used in different types of past-life explorations, and they may be combined with crystals in order to reinforce their efficacy.

The idea behind past-life journeying is that the soul exists outside of time, so the conscious mind is theoretically able to access the soul's history through hypnosis, meditation, or astral travel. Because the soul is too great to fit into a single human experience or incarnation, many lifetimes occur in order to help the soul refine and awaken to remembering its inherent divinity. Along the way, it is possible for certain events to recur and the same people (in reincarnated forms) to keep crossing our paths when our karma with them remains unresolved.

When a pattern repeats frequently in your life and it cannot be understood from an examination of your thoughts or emotions alone, it may often have roots in concurrent lifetimes. In these cases, the causal pattern of the karma in question is creating so much inertia that the cycles will repeat in subsequent incarnations. Past-life regressions can offer a unique perspective on how and why these cycles were born in the first place.

In many instances, merely viewing the events from concurrent lives will allow you to integrate their underlying message. Doing so initiates a process of awakening the soul to the lesson or teaching needed to overcome the karmic inertia. This may result in the end of a karmic pattern in your current incarnation. Sometimes people will experience spontaneous physical healing, attain emotional relief and fulfillment, or enter the next chapter of their spiritual growth by merely engaging in such an experience. Other times seekers will be given enough insight to know how to enact the change on their own. It is possible that the real aim of a past-life journey is to uncover the "why" behind your current state, such that different choices can be made going forward. The karma can be resolved only when it is fully understood. For this reason, past-life regression can open doors that seemed otherwise unavailable to you.

A third option is that merely viewing a past, or future, life is insufficient for creating real and lasting change. In such cases it may be possible to effect change in the past life *at the point of origin*. Although this can be achieved through conventional means of meditation and hypnosis-induced regression, there are a number of crystals that can facilitate the process, too. The benefit of this type of past-life journey is that the participant is not a passive viewer, but an active agent of change.

When past-life journeys reveal traumatic events, it can sometimes feel disempowering to view them. When the journey shifts from passive regression to an active exploration, the person experiencing his or her concurrent lifetime is able to alter the actions taken, thus releasing all subsequent karma. In addition to healing causal patterns retained from other lives, it can serve as a preventative measure, thus removing the karma from the timeline altogether. Because of the gravity of the effects, it is necessary to carefully measure the consequences of any changes made to concurrent lifetimes in this manner.

Profound effects can occur from approaching past-life journeys with the intention of changing your soul's timeline. Although you can fix your current karmic condition, it is also possible to worsen it, as well as the karma of others, especially when attempting to alter a past life from an ego-oriented perspective. Thus it is best to plan an exploratory visit first in order to retrieve as much past-life information as possible. Also, plan to use crystals that will help you shift the karma through altering the timeline in a beneficial manner. The time link crystals are among the best supporters in this area. Diamond and other blueprint-supporting crystals can ensure that the choices and changes reflect the highest expression of your soul's template.

Whenever engaging in a past-life regression of any sort, comfort and relaxation are key to a successful journey. Find a cozy place without any disturbances. Creating sacred space also supports a successful regression; experiment with incense, crystals, candles, and other spiritual tools to facilitate the experience. Always set an intention and invoke adequate protection, as the process of allowing the conscious mind to explore beyond the confines of the physical body can sometimes attract attention from other nonphysical beings, both the helpful and the unhelpful varieties.

Crystals that help to support past-life journeys and the recovery of information from concurrent lives include apophyllite, all types of fossils, dumortierite, crystal skulls, flint, golden beryl, jade, banded opal, time link crystals, record keeper crystals, phantom crystals, serpentine, and wind fossil agate. You can combine any of these crystals with individual stones to guide and provide access to specific lifetimes. See chapter 5 for more details on these guide stones and for instructions on performing a past-life regression on your own.

TRANSMUTING KARMA WITH THE VIOLET FLAME

The seventh ray, described in chapter 2 as being represented by ascended master Portia on the Karmic board, provides the necessary frequencies for altering causal information. As the ray of spiritual alchemy, the violet ray can be used to invoke the ceremonial aspect of the soul for transmuting karmic information. Through this mechanism, negative karma is not simply discarded or wiped away, it is effectively transubstantiated into the energy of merit. Negative karma can therefore be transformed from a deleterious pattern of energy into a vibration that supports spiritual growth and overall wellness.

The violet flame is a manifestation of the violet ray, and it is the primary tool for alchemically raising the consciousness, the universal solvent of spiritual patterns. The violet flame is capable of cutting through any blockage or impediment on all levels of existence. It possesses the characteristics of virtue, moderation, and liberty. The violet flame is easily applied to any limitation or challenge, including karmic patterns.

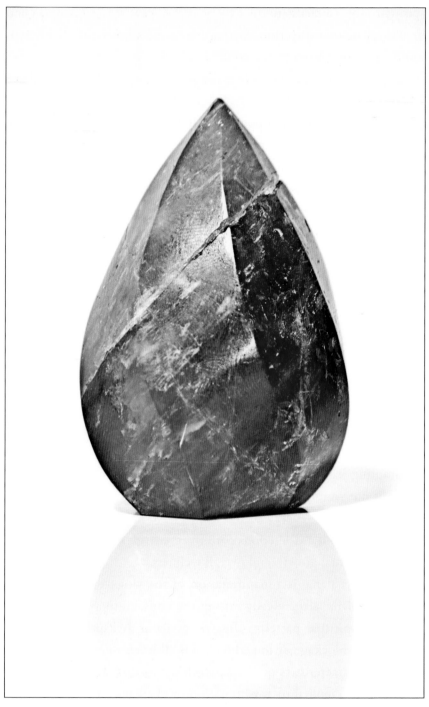

The violet flame

To use the violet flame it is only necessary to visualize purple- or violet-colored flames blazing around the subject of your work. When working on your own karma you can envision this fiery energy covering your physical body and stretching outward to encompass all of the layers of the aura. In this way it will cleanse not only the causal body of negative karma, but it also will resolve karmic energies contained in each level of your being.

The violet flame can be invoked through affirmations or prayers, called *decrees,* as well. Decrees are generally rhythmic and oftentimes rhyming, and many popular decrees have been made available for connecting to the violet flame. Some examples include:

> *I AM a being of violet fire!*
> *I AM the purity God desires![7]*

> *I AM the violet flame*
> *In action in me now*
> *I AM the violet flame*
> *To light alone I bow*
> *I AM the violet flame*
> *In mighty cosmic power*
> *I AM the light of God*
> *Shining every hour*
> *I am the violet flame*
> *Blazing like a sun*
> *I AM God's sacred power*
> *Freeing everyone.[8]*

> *Transmute, transmute by the violet fire all causes*
> *and cores not of God's desire.*
> *I AM a being of cause alone; that cause is Love,*
> *the sacred tone.[9]*

Violet fire burning bright
My causal body is set alight.[10]

These decrees can easily be adapted by altering the words to suit your needs. In the first two examples, "I AM" can be changed to the name of a client, group of people, or nation to employ the violet flame on behalf of others. You are welcome to compose your own or just to speak from the heart when connecting to the power of the flame.

Certain crystals and gemstones can amplify and anchor the potency of the violet flame. Purple- and violet-colored minerals are traditionally associated with the violet flame. Amethyst is the crystalline carrier of the violet ray, and it is therefore the most well-suited gemstone for invoking the violet flame. Other gemstones helpful for karmic release via the violet flame include charoite, purple tourmaline, purple fluorite, purple opal, and Atlantisite. Refer to chapter 5 for specific applications combining the mineral kingdom with the violet flame for healing and transmuting karma.

HEALING PLANETARY KARMA

As the light workers of planet Earth, we are tasked with the special assignment of helping others. The world has entered a critical time during which the human race is being offered a chance to evolve into higher levels of consciousness. The choice to evolve is ours. Collectively, we are nearing the critical mass required for a quantum leap to occur. Since the community of light workers is aware of and actively working toward the next stage in the spiritual progress of the human race, the most proactive step that any one of us can take is to purify and transmute our personal karmic patterns. Each and every particle of your personal karma that is released and healed contributes to the sum total of progress on this planet. If each of us was able to transmute 100 percent of our karma, it is possible that we would be at or near critical mass on a collective scale. However, if there are not enough people working toward this goal, we will never reach the necessary level of karmic release through these methods alone. In light of this, we can partner with one another to achieve healing on a wider scale by compounding our efforts.

Each day brings new opportunities for making decisions; therefore, new aspects of karma are generated by every person on the planet. Leaders of small and large groups of people can make decisions that karmically affect communities and entire nations and even the whole planet. As close as we are to reaching critical mass, it is vitally important to clear collective and planetary karma in addition to our personal karmic debris.

The world is ready for change, and we are on the threshold of experiencing a higher level of consciousness than has ever before been available to humankind. Because of the pressing need to clear out the old in order to make room for the new energies, karmic healing is the most effective means for removing the energetic debris that perpetuates old patterns of thinking and behaving. Each day we can spend several minutes resolving and transmuting planetary karma in order to help ourselves and one another on the path to spiritual realization.

One of the most effective tools for transforming the state of planetary karma is the violet flame. Accordingly, the crystals of the violet ray are excellent implements for accessing and applying the power of the flame. This includes amethyst, the main carrier of the violet ray, as well as charoite, purple tourmaline, purple fluorite, sugilite, lepidolite, violet opal, and other purple gemstones. Other crystals suited to healing planetary karma include diamond, Preseli bluestone, spirit quartz, serpentine, Lemurian seed crystals, the Flame of Ishtar, and Dow crystals. Other stones, such as azurite-malachite and earthkeeper crystals have a special affinity with the entire planet, and they can also help to alleviate the built-up causal energy affecting Earth and all who live on her.

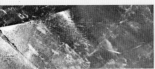
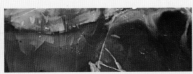
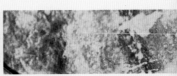

PART 2

✦✦✦

Karmic Stones and How to Use Them

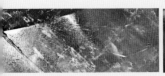
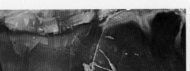
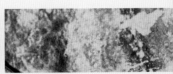

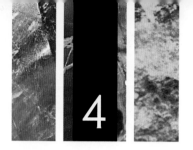

DIRECTORY
OF CRYSTALS
FOR KARMIC HEALING

THE MINERAL KINGDOM is composed of many of the most dynamic healing tools available to humankind. Crystals are direct geometrical expressions of the divine and are thereby endowed with the ability to reach the deepest levels of one's soul for healing. The following stones represent some of the most potent karmic healers I have encountered. Each of these rocks and minerals offers healing by catalyzing spiritual growth, integrating karmic lessons, and otherwise elevating the consciousness in one way or another. Through their application, we can step outside of our karmic limitations and become more crystalline ourselves.

AMAZONITE

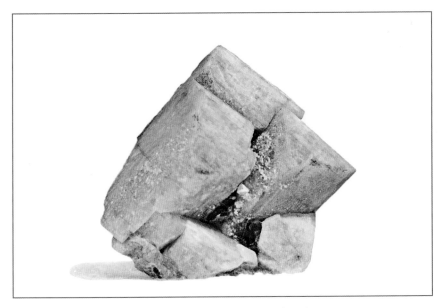

Amazonite crystals from Colorado

Amazonite is a member of the feldspar family that forms in a soft blue or green color. Although its name is derived from the Amazon River, it is more likely to have been so named for its watery color, since no occurrence of greenish feldspar has been found there. Initially, the academic community believed the defining color of amazonite, a blue-to-green shade, was caused by trace amounts of copper. More recent analysis actually points to another metal: lead. Like other minerals that contain lead, it evokes a gentle Saturnian presence for karmic healing.

Amazonite is a stone of speech and truth. It promotes healthy expression by supporting the function of the throat chakra. However, its emphasis is on allowing your actions to be expressions of your highest personal truth. In crystallography the structures of crystals can be classified according to the symmetry of the unit cells; there are seven crystal systems. Amazonite belongs to the triclinic system; its inner axes and outer angles offer the least amount of symmetry of any known crystal group. Amazonite uses this lack of geometrical convention in order to promote stepping out onto your path without judgment; there is no need to "fit in."

Much of the negative karma that we generate is from trying to live someone else's truth or to hide our own in order to please others or meet the needs of society, or simply because we fear the risk of our uniqueness. Amazonite calls in a mild Saturnian influence, since its lead content is so minute; it helps us cultivate the karma of the path that most satisfies the needs of our own spirit. Amazonite is not a stone of transmutation, per se, but it does help to ameliorate karmic ties resulting from not speaking and acting according to your own truth.

Amazonite does not have the high toxicity of many other lead-bearing stones, so it is safe for daily wear or carrying. It sometimes displays a gentle sheen, called a *schiller,* which reminds us that when we live our truth, we truly shine. In doing so, we release worry and attachment, which allows us to bring more joy to the world. As we become conduits of more peace, happiness, and contentment, we accrue merit, or good karma. Amazonite can be a gentle guidepost for following your heart and being in service to the world.

AMETHYST

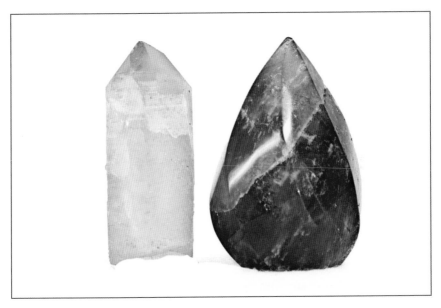

Natural amethyst from Japan (left)
and in the form of polished violet flame (right)

Amethyst is the crystalline anchor for the violet ray on the planet. One of the chief functions of the violet ray is to let go of attachments. Within the context of healing on a causal level, the violet ray can search out and target karmic attachments. These may result from karma in this lifetime or concurrent lives, as well as from family karma inherited at birth. The violet ray serves as a vehicle for releasing and transforming our attachments through a process of alchemy. The primary carrier of this violet energy is amethyst, although some other stones may share its mission in releasing karma.

As the mineral emissary of the violet ray, amethyst embodies the principle of nonattachment as well as carrying out the seventh ray directives of ritual and alchemy. Amethyst is one of the most available healing stones on the planet, and it is a simple tool to use for releasing karma. Simply programming a piece to wear or carry will enable it to focus its transmutational properties on the causal body and our karma.

Amethyst, whose name is derived from Greek for "not drunken," represents abstinence and temperance. Since a goblet carved from amethyst and filled with water would make it appear as though it contained wine, the support of amethyst helps us to refrain from self-destructive and limiting thoughts and behaviors. In this way, this purple quartz guides the person away from generating more negative, harmful karma.

The presence of amethyst is overtly spiritual. It generates a field around it that is calm, serene, and vaguely holy. When amethyst is used for karmic healing, it acts as an invitation for Spirit to take over. This crystal fosters the necessary state of surrender required to engage in truly spiritual living. In this state, we resolve much of our outstanding karma that results from trying to be in control. Alongside this effect, it also supports intuition, meditation, and healing; we just can't help but nourish the soul with amethyst.

The most important function of amethyst as a carrier of the violet ray is in the realm of transmutation. Amethyst acts as a lens, condensing the ray into a particular area. As it focuses this spiritual light, it ignites as the violet flame. The violet flame is one of the most versatile spiritual tools, and it is capable of transforming any disharmonious energy into positivity, including karma itself.

APOPHYLLITE

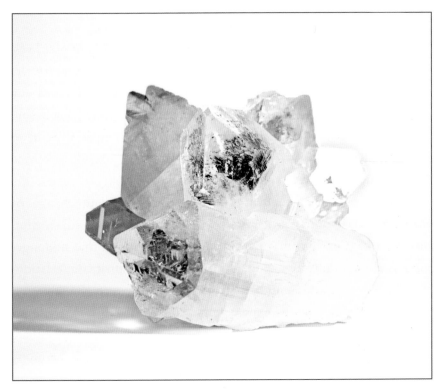

Apophyllite cluster

Apophyllite belongs to the phyllosilicate mineral group and is found worldwide. Although once believed to be a single mineral, its composition varies enough to represent three different and closely related mineral species. It usually occurs in igneous environments, frequently alongside a diverse group of silicate minerals called *zeolites,* with which it shares many qualities. Apophyllite forms pyramid-shaped crystals, and they may be colorless to white, brown, green, pink, or yellow. The specimens are highly prismatic, and when generally free of flaws they appear to glow as if lit from within.

Apophyllite is an insight stone. It brings clarity to the intuition when placed on the third eye, and its tetragonal crystal structure is very stabilizing. This mineral ushers in a sense of brilliance of spirit, and it helps make that accessible by fortifying the etheric body to hold this light. Because it strengthens the etheric body, apophyllite is a great choice for out-of-body travel, such as past-life regressions.

Apophyllite also assists in moving the stagnant energy of past lives, especially by "awakening wisdom and understanding of the past."[1] Its insightful nature furnishes realizations about the karmic level of any scenario. It can bring a flash of comprehension of the underlying lesson, thus permitting release and removal of karma. This is especially true of any limitations or limiting beliefs we carry around as a result of karmic wounds, such as poverty, silence, and chastity.[2]

Use apophyllite in tandem with chrysotile to update, change, or erase soul-level contracts. It can also be coupled with obsidian, flint, or black phantom selenite to cut through ties of karma that no longer serve your growth. Green apophyllite is able to illuminate our relationship with money and abundance, which can really turn the tables on previous karmic patterns in these areas. Apophyllite clusters are luminous tools for scrubbing the etheric and causal bodies, and they radiate their light into the surrounding room. They promote family harmony and heal wounds and rifts among family members that are leftover from previous lifetimes.

AQUAMARINE

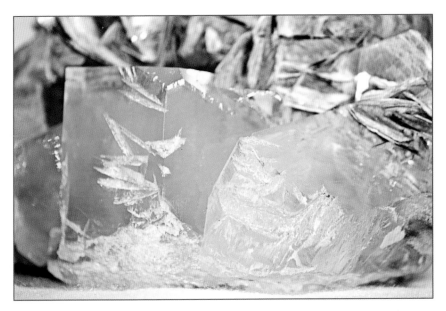

Aquamarine invokes images of water and release.

When beryl contains iron and shows a blue-to-green color it is called *aquamarine,* a name that comes from the Latin for "seawater" because of its characteristic hue. Aquamarine is a perennial favorite among gemstones for its attractive color and good durability. In its natural state aquamarine crystallizes as hexagonal prisms, and it may on occasion occur in tandem with heliodor.

Aquamarine is a stone of release. It teaches the benefit of going with the flow and brings light and clarity to any condition. Frequently used for inspiration, creativity, and expression, aquamarine can also help us to see the bigger picture in terms of cyclical patterns. Just like the ocean's tides, all of creation has an ebb and flow. Aquamarine harmonizes its wearer with these rhythms.

Aquamarine is a capable cleanser; like bathing in ocean water, aquamarine's energy soothes old wounds of the mind, body, and soul. It deeply relaxes the body and awakens a higher awareness at the same time. Together, this makes for the ideal state for performing causal healing. Its detoxifying properties work predominantly at the physical level, and over time aquamarine extends its reach to all levels of our beings. This crystal sheds light on the stuck, crystallized patterns deeply embedded in the soul and psyche in order to alleviate the stress and pain of the scenario.

The morphology of beryl holds a geometrical key to its connection to the blueprint level. While aquamarine's external crystal is hexagonal, x-ray diffraction reveals that its molecules align perfectly with the template of creation, the Flower of Life. The Flower of Life is the original blueprint for creation; as such, it strongly connects us to our personal blueprint in order to clear out any residue or baggage that may be preventing the inherent order and divinity of our blueprint from shining through to express itself. Although all forms of beryl contain this same physical template, aquamarine appears to connect more deeply than other beryls to the spiritual blueprint.

Simultaneously, the watery character that aquamarine confers promotes a state of fluidity, which has been described as "energetic liquidity."[3] This liquidity enables states of manifest reality at any level of organization—from our tiniest components to our whole being—to move between the manifest form and the premanifest state. This process is similar to how photons, the base unit of light, can be either particles (a more or less physical structure) or waves (a fluid-like energy). By restoring the ability to resume a state of liquidity, our manifest forms—whether they are physical, mental, or emotional—can revert to an energetic state that enables them to communicate clearly with their spiritual blueprint. Being able to regain this means of communication permits manifest patterns to correct their courses, thereby responding in time to causal energies as they take place.

Aquamarine is one of few crystals that conveys a deep relationship with the blueprint of our existence. Because of this, it harmonizes well with diamond and trigonic quartz. Aquamarine can be used to prime the pump for other forms of karmic healing by engendering greater fluidity. It is a versatile gem with many applications, and it is a valuable addition to any healer's toolbox.

CARNELIAN

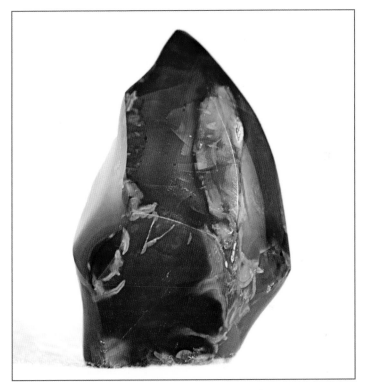

A polished carnelian flame from Madagascar

Carnelian is a member of the quartz family; specifically, it is an orange-colored agate, whose color is derived from iron. Although the most sought-after carnelian is a true orange, natural carnelian varies from brown and red through all shades of orange and yellow. Occasionally it may occur with transparent, pink, or other colored patches, too.

The mission of carnelian is to offer support through vitality. Using carnelian can offer a boost of energy, stimulate the metabolism, and help to inspire happiness and optimism. Carnelian has been a popular gem for millennia, and traditional resources often ascribe to it a protective influence. Older sources also commonly describe this gemstone as conferring success and courage.

Using carnelian for causal-level healing inspires change through action. Carnelian can be used to break out of tiresome karmic patterns and self-destructive habits because it grants a step up into a more positive frame of mind. These qualities supersede the effects of karmic baggage, and they often displace the visible effects of karma in our current scenario. At the causal level, carnelian's action improves the fundamental patterning that underpins any karmic cycle. By changing the basic fabric of causal reality, negative emotional patterns, behaviors, and physical conditions can also change. This helps to resolve the influence that past decisions continue to exert in our daily lives.

Carnelian offers a favorable push toward success in any endeavor. It is helpful to use in tandem with other karmic healing stones when it appears as though progress is stagnating. Not only will it contribute to getting things jump-started, carnelian will also inspire a more optimistic attitude, thereby leveling the playing field on two fronts at once.

CERUSSITE

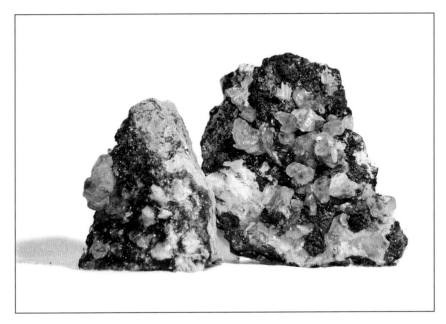

Cerussite

Cerussite is a common ore of lead that occurs through the weathering of other lead minerals. It is generally white or colorless, although trace amounts of other minerals can result in gray, blue, or green crystals. It is frequently twinned, a phenomenon that occurs when two separate crystals share some of the same crystal lattice points in a symmetrical manner, resulting in an intergrowth of two separate crystals in a variety of specific configurations. This twinning allows it to superficially resemble snowflakes. Cerussite was once used as the chief pigment of white, lead-based paints and cosmetics. Since this can yield toxic products, their use has been largely abandoned. Cerussite is generally safe to handle, but care should be taken so as to limit exposure. It may be safely carried in a pouch, used in a crystal grid, or made into an elixir by indirect methods; ***never ingest cerussite.***

Cerussite, for its lead content and high specific gravity, is an effective grounding tool. It helps us maintain a sense of brightness and spiritual lightness while being fully aware and fully embodied here in the third dimension. It is thus helpful for people who have a hard time fitting in on Earth, either because their souls are from other places or planes, or because of the amount of karma, suffering, and pain that exists on Earth. Cerussite acts like a web of light that courses its way through our physical and nonphysical anatomies. It helps to activate the nervous system, and it can be used to treat disorders associated therewith.

Cerussite has a penchant for identifying those people with whom you've shared past lives.[4] In its cyclic twin form, which is star-like in appearance, it can help you contact your past incarnations that may have occurred off-world. It also triggers the appearance and visualization of threads of karmic energy that bind and connect souls that have shared lifetimes. This can highlight opportunities to apply other crystals for releasing karma and for healing long-held wounds. Cerussite, as a lead crystal, also connects us to the energy of Saturn for karmic healing.

CHAROITE

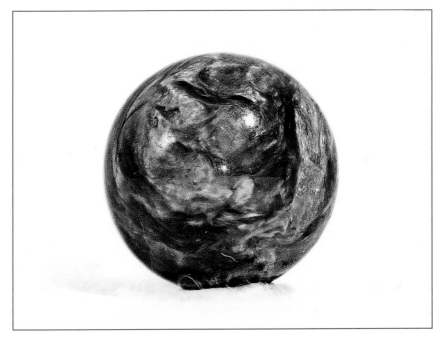

A polished charoite exhibits enchanting purple swirls.

Charoite is a purple gem from Russia formed by metamorphic processes. It has a pronounced velvety shimmer from the broken and twisted fibrous crystals within. Charoite helps us ground spiritual purpose into every action we take. It enables you to find greater security when traveling your path. This gemstone promotes insight during the dream state, objectivity with regard to intuitive information, and connection to the unconscious mind.

The chatoyant, swirling pattern in charoite represents the movement of the inner self. The mind can be just as tumultuous and tempestuous as its fibers. Thanks to the violet ray, this stone calls in the power of identifying and releasing limitations in order to target fears and feelings of inadequacy in the subconscious. As these latent mental and emotional energies are brought to light, they can be consciously transformed and healed.

Overall, the mission of charoite is to facilitate finding a way to be of service to others.[5] The manganese content of this metamorphic rock, which endows it with its purple hue, is an activator of the heart center. Charoite unifies our spiritual direction with what brings us the greatest amount of joy. Through service we are better able to spread love, healing, and wholeness to the world. Allowing yourself to accomplish your path of service is an act of merit, and it generates more positive karma. Charoite can balance karma's scales in favor of your soul by releasing and transmuting negative karma while simultaneously aligning you with the path of service to others.

Charoite has a refining effect on the body, as it helps the spiritual ideal to be welcomed into the physical plane. It especially integrates the physical aspect of our spiritual bodies "into a perfect crystalline structure that allows you a clear connection with your soul and brings its full participation into your life."[6] Charoite is most helpful in this avenue when used as an elixir and coupled with clear quartz, "as it clarifies even more the ideal [or blueprint] for human DNA and helps the cells use it in rebuilding your bodily structure during transformation."[7]

CRYSTAL SKULLS

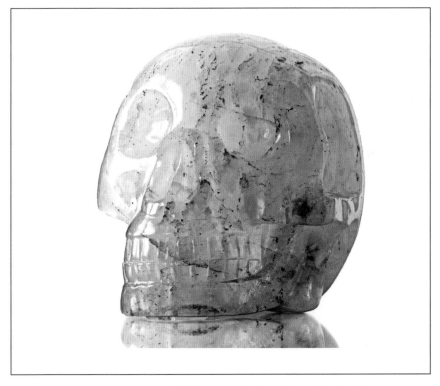

Mustang, an ancient skull from Nepal; from the author's collection

Among today's crystal lovers, crystal skulls are popular tools for healing and meditation. Many different styles are carved by modern lapidary artists, and many different kinds of crystals and gemstones are used to make them. Ancient skulls can be found in various places, especially in the Americas, China, Tibet, Mongolia, Nepal, and occasionally in Europe. More recently made skulls work equally well for our purposes of karmic release.

The energy of a crystal skull works on a collective level. The skull is a universal symbol for humankind, and it reminds one that beneath every face is a skull so similar as to be difficult to identify who is who without rigorous training. This energy of unity begets a sense of wonderment and compassion, both of which can instigate compassionate action for accomplishing meritorious acts. In this way, crystal skulls can anchor a new wave of positive transformation and the generation of good karma.

Since they depict the human cranium, crystal skulls have an inherently mental association. These crystalline tools offer clarity to the mind and mental bodies. A number of different crystalline substances are used in the technological industry as a means of storing data, and quartz crystal skulls can be used with similar effects on a spiritual level. Accessing crystal-skull consciousness reveals our soul's memories, which often relate to our current karmic conditions. The light and crystallinity that are intrinsic characteristics of crystal skulls will align, illumine, and erase stored karmic memories.

Crystal skulls are often linked to planetary changes and the consciousness of all denizens of Earth. The skulls are noted for their collective consciousness, which spreads around the globe in a grid or net of light from the skulls' positions all over the world. In light of this, crystal skulls are excellent tools for healing planetary karma, too. Combine them with other planetary or genealogical healing stones in order to focus their energy on a bigger scale. When coupled with karmic resolvers such as opals, amethyst, or time link crystals, the effects are greatly accelerated.

DIAMOND

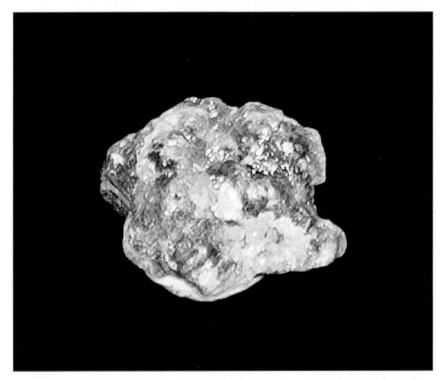

Raw diamond crystal

Diamonds are crystalline carbon, famed for their role in the gem-stone industry. Diamonds exhibit extraordinary brilliance, toughness, and clarity. They are cubic minerals and grow in a multitude of crystal forms. Diamonds have been favored as talismans for millennia for their unbeatable hardness and their inner and outer perfection.

Diamond is the principal healer of the blueprint. It expresses its own blueprint's inherent perfection with such conviction that it can influence others to do the same.[8] In ancient writings, diamonds are described as the invincible gems that can cut through illusion, dark-ness, and danger in order to permit the qualities of light and healing to shine through. Diamonds similarly cut through our karmic conditions. They sever them at the source, which lies in our spiritual blueprint. The diamond offers extreme transformation at the blueprint level, which may be profound, if not sometimes tumultuous. The diamond can be used on its own, especially when employing diamonds of unparalleled clarity and brilliance. Raw, unpolished diamonds have much more diffuse effects, and they can safely be used when effectively cleansed and cleared beforehand.

To use diamonds in karmic healing they should be placed on the third eye or the heart, or they may be held over the causal chakra. Diamond's effects are generally quite strong, so it is necessary to exercise sensitivity and caution when applying them therapeutically. To offer a gentler experience when accessing diamond's ability to clear the blueprint, try using it in tandem with grounding stones such as hematite or magnetite, as well as softening crystals like rose quartz, aventurine, or rhodonite.

Diamond also has a reputation of cutting through limitation and illusion so dynamically that it is often associated with the symbolism of the thunderbolt in traditional spiritual literature. In Buddhist and Hindu texts the word for diamond is the same as the word for thunderbolt; it equates to the brilliance and expediency of the flash of enlightenment. This is the same manner in which diamond works on our blueprint. We cannot achieve enlightenment when we carry too much karmic baggage, so diamond clears and aligns our blueprint with Source, thereby enabling us to ready ourselves for the next chapter in our spiritual evolution.

DUMORTIERITE

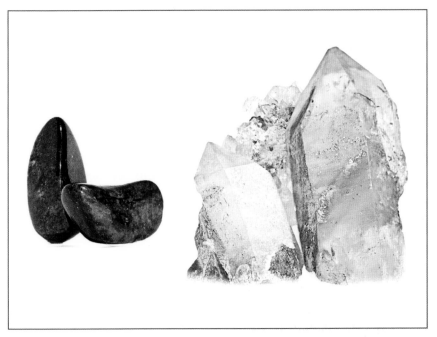

Polished dumortierite (left) and dumortierite inclusions in quartz

Dumortierite is a silicate of aluminum, and it is usually found in the blue-to-violet spectrum. Its rich indigo hue is derived from traces of zinc, manganese, and iron, and it is also found as needle-like or fibrous inclusions in massive quartz, coloring it blue (called aventurine, in this case). Overall, the effect of dumortierite is pacifying. It promotes relaxation and fosters tolerance. Dumortierite offers an integration of memories from the soul; placing it on the past-life chakras can facilitate recall of past-life memories.[9] It is especially helpful in understanding soul contracts because it guides you to the inception of your soul's journey and the subsequent agreements made along in its development.[10] It can also be used to consciously break through any of these limiting beliefs and agreements.

Dumortierite is the stone of patience, for it invites us to find stillness and peace at every step of our path.[11] This results in a positive attitude, better communication, and greater trust. It is an excellent stone for living in the now because it helps to release the expectations and attachments to outcomes that are so tremendously ingrained in modern thinking. Dumortierite can also facilitate a Saturnian awareness of cycles, thanks to its indigo color, but it does so without being a victim of linear time. This gemstone brings a sense of peace that overpowers the ticking of the clock, thereby freeing the soul to live in a comfortable and natural temporal cycle. Dumortierite can therefore instill an awareness of compulsive patterns as well as help to dissolve them.[12] It will help to release these patterns from our causal body, thus freeing one from the karma built up around them.

FLAME OF ISHTAR

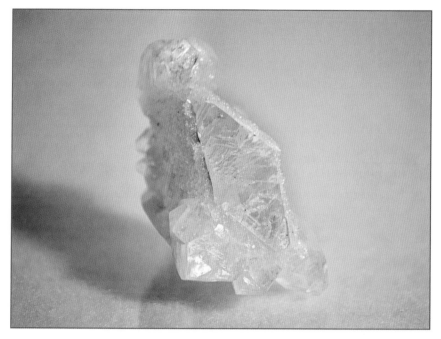

Flame of Ishtar

The Flame of Ishtar is an unusual configuration of apophyllite with a calcite core, discovered and named by lapidary artist and jeweler Bob Geisel.[13] Occasionally when apophyllite is cut and polished it will reveal a rhombus-shaped interior of white or clear calcite; this is the Flame of Ishtar. These configurations are not easy to find, but they will seek out their new owners in the right timing.

The Flame of Ishtar acts as a doorway to higher realms of consciousness, a portal to assist evolution and spiritual transformation. The apophyllite itself is often used for facilitating astral travel and psychic abilities. These energies guide and direct the flame to the realm of the higher mind, enabling the stone to grant immediate access to our spiritual mind. Because of this, they can be used to journey to the Akashic records in order to promote spiritual learning, including the understanding of past lives and karmic patterns.

Named for the Mesopotamian goddess of the heavenly realms, these special crystal formations manifest her celestial hope, innate wisdom, and guiding light. The inner rhombus of calcite possesses calcite's ability to link parallel realities, thereby conferring the skill to pass from one dimension or reality into another. This inner doorway is shaped with remarkable symmetry, and its diamond-like appearance is a representation of the spiritual axiom "As above, so below." White calcite also bestows karmic grace by detoxifying patterns not in harmony with your soul's blueprint.

The luminous, fiery nature of the Flame of Ishtar is highly purifying. It can burn through the dross of mental and emotional baggage, spiritual doubt, and even our negative karma while also pushing away fear. The "above" represented in the inner doorway is perfection in its most absolute form. Since we are meant to recognize and reclaim our inner, immanent divinity, the Flame of Ishtar helps to manifest this cosmic perfection here on the Earth plane. The flame, especially given its apophyllite content, therefore helps to promote alignment with our blueprint; such a "Divine Alignment means coming into healthy relationship with the divine plan that your soul or higher self has agreed to honour [in] this lifetime."[14] It is one of the critical stones that has appeared during this most pivotal time in the unfoldment of human consciousness.

FLINT

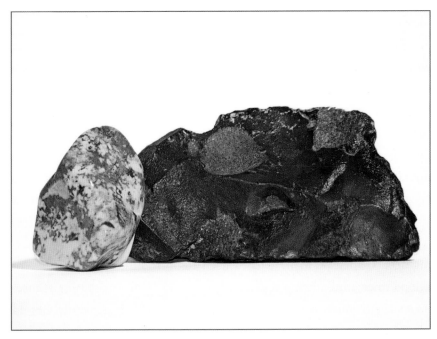

Rough flint from Florida and polished specimen from Flint Ridge, Ohio

A variety of chert, flint is composed of tiny grains of quartz that form as a replacement of calcium carbonate in chalk and limestone. Once revered by ancient people, flint's utility in sparking fires and its aptitude for cutting made it a valuable commodity. Legends surrounding flint arose, and it was often linked to otherworldly beings, such as the fairy folk and the gods. Wearing or carrying flint was often done to prevent these beings from interfering in life as well as for connecting to their power for good use.

Flint represents a connection between worlds. Folklore indicates that it was often placed above the doorway for protection, indicating an association with liminal zones, the thresholds between realities. Fine pieces of flint often have a ringing quality; they are resonant when struck. This resonance acts like a beacon to help one move between realities and journey in time. For this reason, flint makes an excellent journeying stone when working to revisit previous lifetimes in order to glean a clearer idea of how and why they are affecting one's present incarnation.

The ability to cross realities also enables flint to facilitate contact with other levels of consciousness. Tradition dictates that flint has a long-standing connection to the realms of the fairies, who are the embodiments of the consciousness of nature, as well as to the ancestors.[15] Meditating with flint can open the doorway to accessing the intelligence of these realms; many of these beings are willing to help humanity with their evolution, including the release of karma. The ancestral energy carried by flint permits it to be one of the stones best attuned to healing genealogical karma.

Because flint is often available with sharp edges even without having been shaped by man, it lends itself to auric surgery. Flint is one of the premier cord-cutting tools, and its attunement across time focuses its specialty onto cords from previous lifetimes. It is generally viewed as a purifying stone, too, helping to tease out attachments lodged in the chakras and various layers of the aura. It can be raked or combed through the aura to detect and dislodge foreign energies and past-life attachments.

Flint is a fiery and earthy member of the quartz clan. Using it can promote stability, helping to root you more fully in the present moment. Flint's timelessness and liminal focus allow one to remain centered and aware of the eternal Now. Since flint has long been used to ignite fires, it can also be a stone of action. When absolutely necessary, flint is always ready to spark the fire of action, catalyzing the movement necessary to step closer into wholeness.

FOSSILS

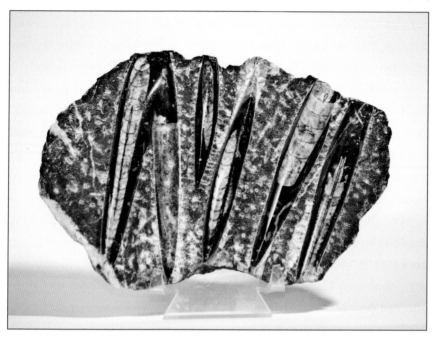

Orthoceras fossils from Morocco

Fossils occur in one of two ways: they are either a mineral replacement of organic material or they may be casts and imprints of living material. Fossils occur around the world, and they range in age from very, very ancient to relatively recent. Quartz is frequently the cause of the mineralization process, although many other substances can perform the same function. Common fossilized minerals include fossilized algae (stromatolite), bones and teeth, plant matter, shells and exoskeletons, and numerous other remnants of the past.

Generally speaking, fossils were some of the earliest sacred stones used by our ancient forebears. They bridge the living and the nonliving. They were once animals or plants and now are suspended in time as stones. All fossils are believed to confer protection, longevity, and a connection to the natural world. Fossils as a whole may also be used for connecting to past lives and clearing karma. These stones also represent eternity and evolution; connecting to them is helpful for releasing old programming and for maintaining a sense of calm in a state of crisis.

As sedimentary stones, fossils help to sift through the debris and baggage that we carry. This makes them helpful for resolving karma, especially that which is stored in the causal body. The causal body is composed of bands and layers reminiscent of sedimentary rock, thus making fossils attuned to sorting through and stabilizing the information of the causal body. Fossils are traditionally connected to the past, since they are the product of the passage of time. They serve to provide a window into other eras, such as by connecting to ancestral energy or for undertaking past-life journeys.

Fossils emit a fundamentally Saturnian energy since they preserve only the structure and form in a very skeletal way. The teeth and bones are ruled by this planet, and many fossils are exactly that. Meditating with fossilized bone and fossilized teeth invokes the help of Saturn and can provide insight into the causal patterns of current scenarios. Saturn's influence also emphasizes grounding and impartiality, such that fossils facilitate being an objective observer while assimilating karmic lessons from the past. In addition to the properties listed above, specific qualities are detailed below for the following fossils.

Amber

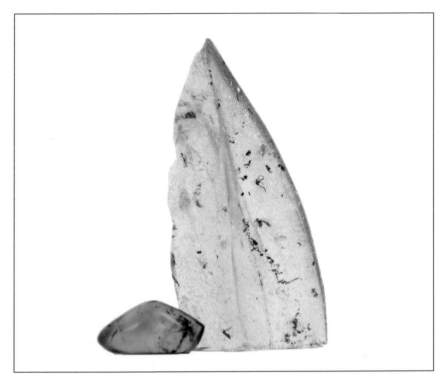

Golden amber from the Dominican Republic
and blue amber from Indonesia

Amber is not a proper fossil since it is still organic in composition, being solidified tree resin that has not undergone complete mineralization. For this reason, amber is also noncrystalline and is not properly considered a mineral. It is found in several locations worldwide, including along the shores of the Baltic Sea, in the Dominican Republic, and in Indonesia. It often contains remnants of plants, insects, and occasionally frogs and lizards preserved within its golden body.

Amber is enlivening and electric. It spreads warmth and cheer wherever it is placed. Amber has the ability to slow time down, which enables one to change course or stop the accumulation of karma from a specific instance altogether. Just as amber suspends ancient plants and creatures within its core, this gem can further your understanding of the karmic implications of any thought, action, or intention by suspending it in the mind. This permits you to examine it from all angles before carrying through. Amber can be helpful for indecision, because it allows one to reach a state of certainty before acting.

Amber feels like drops of solidified sunlight. In fact, since plants convert sunlight into their own food and energy supplies, the resin that would become amber is akin to the transport for said fuel. Amber actually is solar light made solid! It can bring this solar energy to stagnant areas of life, including stale karmic patterns. It supports success, charisma, and joy in all endeavors. Since it is still organic, it has a strong resonance with the organic makeup of our bodies. It can condense and highlight its energy on the cellular memories in our DNA; combine it with a purifying stone such as shungite to clean out the imprint of negative karma from the genetic level of your being.

Ammonite

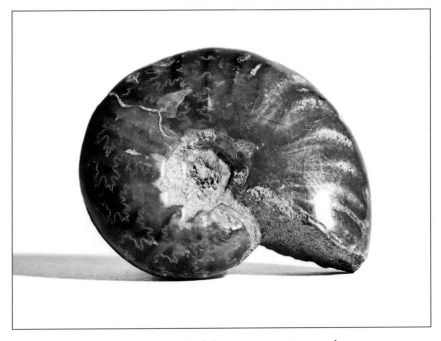

An ammonite fossil shows an attractive spiral.

Ammonite is the fossilized spiral shell of an invertebrate that resembles the modern-day nautilus. Ammonite fossils display a beautiful spiral pattern when polished. These fossils link us to the cyclical nature of time. Often the logical mind rationalizes the passage of time in a purely linear fashion. The spiritual reality of time is that it is entirely concurrent; only the earthly part of our entire existence perceives it as linear.

Ammonites are portal stones; they can open doorways to other times and other planes of consciousness. They make excellent crystals to accompany you on past-life regression, and they may also be used to explore future lives. Ammonites can be placed on the body in order to help break free from an illness or injury resulting from the repetition of a karmic cycle. Working with ammonite fossils opens the doorway to understanding why karma repeats, as they can shed light on the initial karmic event that set the patterns in motion.

Calcitized Shells

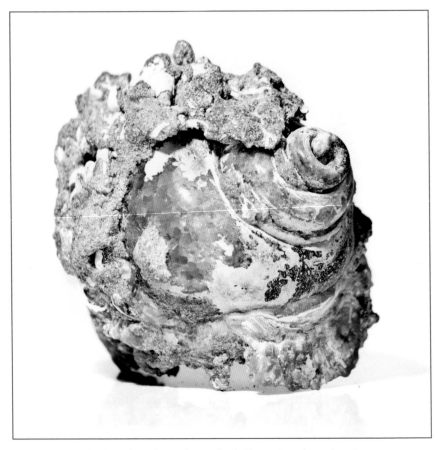

Shells such as this calcitized whelk are found in Florida.

Calcitized shells are fossils found mostly in Florida. The calcium carbonate in the shells is converted to golden calcite as the shells metamorphose into fossils. The calcites are typically a medium-to-pale shade of gold and will fluoresce under ultraviolet light. Calcite exhibits perfect cleavage in three directions and will cleave into perfect rhombohedral forms. Calcite is abundant worldwide, and it is one of the prevalent crystals for ushering in higher consciousness to Earth.

Calcitized fossil shells bring the delightful, almost tropical combination of sand, sun, and sea into crystalline form. They perfectly embody the energy of my home state, and holding these crystals can almost conjure a refreshing sea breeze. Because of their crystalline calcite, these fossils have a loftier energy than most other fossils. They are very uplifting.

The energy of golden calcite promotes centeredness and awareness of the present moment. In connecting to golden calcite we are empowered to make changes and to apply the presence of mind to evolve with courage and joy. These special fossils channel the spontaneous, golden ray of calcite into the causal level. Meditating with them can facilitate breaking free from patterns in which we are stubbornly fixed. When karmic patterns have too much momentum to change course, even as we begin to assimilate their lessons, these fossilized shells can offer much-needed freedom and change.

The rhombohedral units in which calcite forms help to link parallel realities.[16] This property can be harnessed for accessing higher realms of consciousness such as the causal plane or for experiencing concurrent lifetimes in order to learn and grow. Calcite possesses a means of uniting denser and more spiritual realities. Working with it provides traction and healing, especially when combined with other karmic stones. Try using it with flint to journey to past lives connected to the ocean.

Fossilized Coral

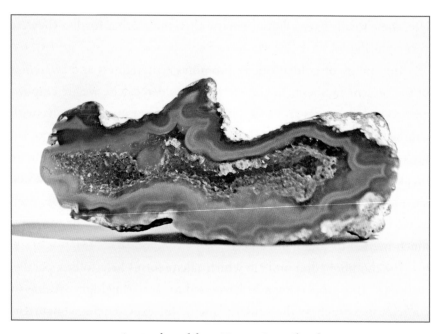

Agatized coral from Tampa Bay, Florida

Fossilized coral occurs in many places worldwide, in a number of different configurations. It may be agatized or calcitized, and accessory minerals can offer stunning displays of color. Some famous deposits of coral fossils are found around Lake Michigan, in several parts of Florida, in Indonesia, and other places. Many different species of coral can be fossilized, offering a wide variety of gemstones.

Coral is composed of the skeletons of millions of tiny organisms that live in marine environments as a single colony. They create their colony out of calcium carbonate, and it builds slowly as new coral polyps build on the exoskeletons of their predecessors. When fossilized, these gemstones continue to emphasize the quality of building on what has been left behind. Fossilized coral is perfect for listening to the voices of our ancestors, for guidance, or for healing, as well as for connecting to the family identity. Coral polyps in a single mass are usually genetically identical, which reminds us to focus on the underlying oneness in all life.

Fossilized coral may be best suited for healing the karma of a community. This can include genealogical karma, which is the karma of the family community over eons; however, it can also be applied to other concepts of community, too. For example, adding coral to your crystal grids can allow it to heal the karma of a town, organization, or nation. It can also help to offer support by looking for the lineage or tradition that drives and motivates communities toward growth.

The action of fossilized coral, when used for healing karma, is not immediately directed at karmic release. Instead, it reaches through all the individuals in the targeted group and awakens the recognition of oneness at a basic, almost cellular level. It revives the connection to the realm of the ancestors and reminds each person that we do not have to feel alone. Not only are we surrounded by others who can come together to support one another in communities, but we also have the assistance and guidance of all those who have come before us. In doing so, we can consciously choose to let go of the old weight of karma building up on our shoulders.

Many coral polyps typically exhibit a sixfold symmetry. When polished, some types of fossilized colony corals will portray the same morphology, which activates a deeply longed-for love in every cell of the body. In numerology, six is the vibration of love, and it also unites Heaven and Earth for co-creation. Coral, in fossil form, helps to form a bridge between realities and planes of existence. It connects the living with the nonliving, animal with mineral, sea with stone, Heaven with Earth. It is a powerful ally in building a new global community free from the limitations of our previous choices.

Fossilized Teeth

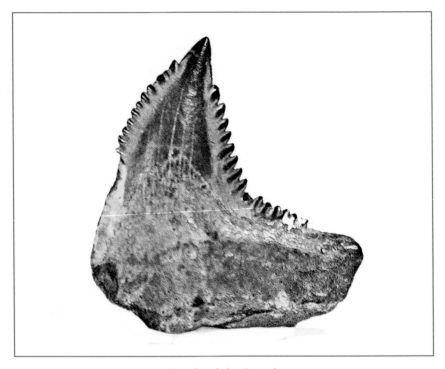

Fossilized shark tooth

Beaches around the world are awash in the fossilized remains of sharks. Since these creatures are cartilaginous fish, only their teeth are calcified, making them the most apt parts of their anatomy to fossilize. The teeth of other vertebrates may also be found in fossil beds worldwide, including the teeth of horses, dinosaurs, fish, and numerous other creatures.

Fossilized teeth can help break karmic patterns associated with speech. When the soul is stunted through lack of communication, a pattern can build, yielding lifetimes of timidity, shyness, and a fear of intimate expression. Tooth fossils can embolden the ability to express oneself in order to step out of a karmic rut. The teeth often represent your ability to defend yourself, and these fossils contribute to standing up for yourself by making your voice heard.

The remains of predatory organisms such as sharks' teeth are adequate tools for cord-cutting rituals, too. Their innate sharpness cuts through limitations and fears as easily as energetic cords. Use them to support your ability to seize the moment and to find the right timing for expressing yourself.

Petrified Wood

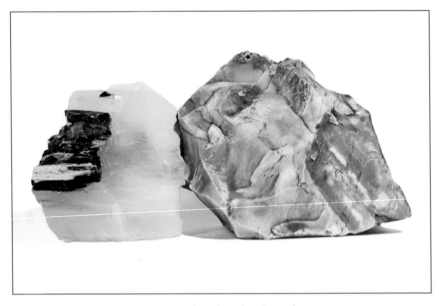

Agatized and opalized wood

Petrified wood is easily the most abundant fossil in crystal shops today. It is found in many places worldwide, and there are instances of entire forests surviving in petrified form. Most petrified wood is a silica replacement and can be more specifically termed *agatized wood;* many other minerals can also yield wood fossils, including pyrite, calcite, opal, and others. Various trace elements result in the variety of colors in which petrified wood is found.

A stone of new beginnings, petrified wood makes opportunists out of us all. When some cataclysm ended the life of the tree from which this fossil is derived, the tree easily could have been broken down, eaten away by microorganisms, or otherwise lost to the sands of time. However, when all the conditions are just right, the organic material in the wood is replaced by silica or other minerals. Petrified wood defies the odds and does more than survive; it literally crystallizes under immense stress and becomes more durable and beautiful than ever.

Petrified wood opens the eyes to perceive obstacles as opportunities and challenges as a chance to make a change. On a karmic level this means that petrified wood redirects karmic patterns into advantageous routes. As you use it in your healing practice, petrified wood encourages you to accept circumstances for what they are while framing them in a new light. Rather than merely being buried in a landslide or earthquake, the prefossilized tree didn't stop to have a panic attack; instead, the tree surrendered to the process in order to be reborn.

Of all fossils, petrified wood is among the most grounding. It can be used on the base chakra, on the legs, or below the feet to invite the energy field to profoundly connect to the Earth Mother. Doing so helps one truly concede to the overwhelming support always available. It is a useful anchor and guide on past-life journeys, and it makes a wonderful partner with flint or the time link crystals.

GABBRO

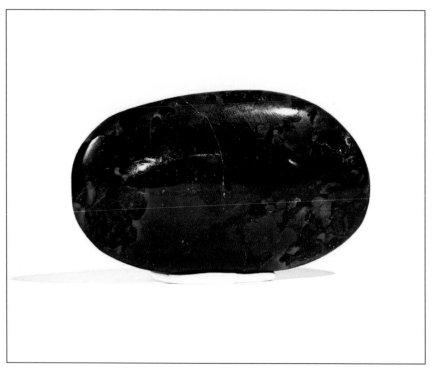

Indigo gabbro from Madagascar

Gabbro is an igneous rock with large or coarse-grained crystals. It is typically composed of feldspar, pyroxene, amphibole, and olivine, as well as accessory minerals. Most gabbro is dark in color, such as black to green, and a few deposits exhibit striking color contrast, such as indigo gabbro (sometimes called mystic merlinite) and blizzard stone.

All gabbro is strongly grounding due to its mineral content. It is rich in heavier metals, which offer support and strength to anyone who holds it. Gabbro can assist in releasing slow-moving energy or illness, as it formed very slowly within Earth's crust. This applies to karmic conditions, too, where it can help latent karma come to a head in order to be dealt with head-on. Blizzard stone, a black-and-white variety of this stone found in Alaska, is exceptionally well-attuned to exposing latent patterns and energies. It can help to illumine repressed karma at the family and community levels in order to help people cope with these causal energies.

Indigo gabbro is my favorite type of gabbro for karmic clearing. It helps to bridge worlds, and it also works closely with the gemstone carriers of the indigo ray. Indigo gabbro shines light into the unconscious mind. It is an apt healing stone, one that is willing to assist in healing conditions of every level of our reality. It opens doorways for the indigo ray energy, and therefore the qualities of Saturn, to sweep through each layer of our aura. The energy of indigo gabbro helps to bring stability and comprehension to the causal layer of our aura, which enables understanding of the "why" behind karma.

Indigo gabbro may facilitate the process of soul retrieval; on past-life excursions one may find these fragmented pieces of the soul that have been severed when certain karma was incurred. Indigo gabbro can help these soul fragments rejoin the body of the individual soul, thereby correcting the expression of the blueprint's intrinsic perfection. To facilitate this process, partner gabbro with stones that help to locate and call the missing pieces of the soul, like rainbow obsidian, astrophyllite, and nuummite. Afterward, sweep through the aura with chrysotile or flint to cleanse the karma that these soul fragments may have been carrying.

GALENA

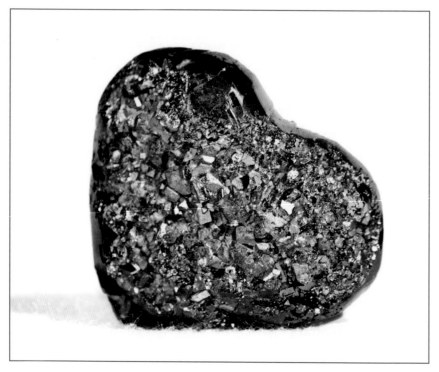

Galena

Lead minerals are important to karmic work, since lead is the metal ruled by Saturn. Of the lead minerals, galena is one of the most available and recognizable. It is a cubic sulfide of lead, and its crystals have a grayish metallic luster. ***Exercise caution with galena;*** while it is safe to handle, inhalation or ingestion of galena dust can be problematic. Limit your exposure and only prepare elixirs via indirect methods.

Lead has a dampening, congealing effect. In a pure state it is very soft and is not a very resonant metal.[17] Each of its ores conveys a similar property, with galena being one of the strongest purveyors of this softening or freezing effect. Lead is not resonant, and it is not likely to form soluble compounds, unlike most other metals. Thus lead— and therefore galena—tends to have an isolating effect; it can focus its energy on a particular aspect or pattern and hold it in place for examination. This can be applied to karmic resolution by holding a causal pattern or aspect of karma in place so it can be seen from all angles without continuing to move forward. This helps to provide better insight before acting to resolve the karma in question.

Galena stimulates looking at life through the lens of karma. It can trigger a causal awareness in the use of intuition, astrology, and scrying.[18] Galena allows you to interpret the events depicted in terms of karmic language and understanding, which can reveal the larger cycles and sequences at work.

HELIODOR (GOLDEN BERYL)

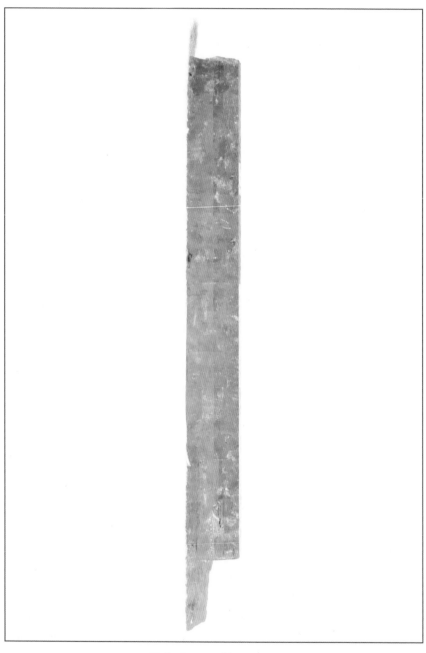

*Heliodor, a golden cousin
to aquamarine and emerald*

Heliodor, named for its cheerful solar color, describes a member of the beryl family. It is yellow to greenish-yellow, and the golden shades are the most desirable for causal healing. Golden beryl works to nourish and support the causal body, as well as offering support to the solar plexus and crown centers. Traditional uses for golden beryl include digestive conditions and lack of vitality. Beryl was often the stone of choice for crystal balls, too.

Golden beryl brings the golden ray into the energy field. The golden ray links us directly to Source, specifically as the Great Central Sun, as explained in the ascended master, I AM teachings. This overtly solar energy vitalizes our sense of power, helping to align personal power with the greater good. On the causal level, this feature helps to overcome past-life scenarios resulting in a loss of power today. Golden beryl can be applied to restore the right use of power, especially when karma ties to lifetimes such as that of Atlantis, wherein power was greatly abused to the detriment of everyone, and it can therefore encourage one to step gently into a position of decisive action.

Golden beryl ushers a brilliant light into the causal body. It first activates and empowers the stellar gateway chakra, one of the transpersonal chakras located approximately one foot above the crown; following this, its energy moves through the soul star chakra and into the crown chakra. Consciously directing it to link the stellar gateway with the causal chakra, located behind and below the crown, sheds light on the law of cause and effect that governs the universe. As the energy of heliodor moves into the energy field, it focuses its efforts at the causal layer of the aura.

Golden beryl strengthens and tones the causal body with its nourishing light. As it offers its support, the function of memory and recall is stimulated in the causal body within the aura. Regularly working with or wearing golden beryl can offer improved memory, both long-term and short-term.[19] At first this may result in random, unexpected glimmers of memory. It is helpful to couple its efforts with more stabilizing gemstones, which will steady the action on the memory and prevent unwanted flashes.

Combined with a past-life stone such as flint, golden beryl is able to better focus the effect of traveling to experience the source of our karma. Flint will open the portal, and heliodor will magnify and clarify the journey altogether. Golden beryl also pairs well with any stones that target karmic release, since the nourishing and strengthening of the causal body makes it more resilient during healing and letting go.[20]

JADE

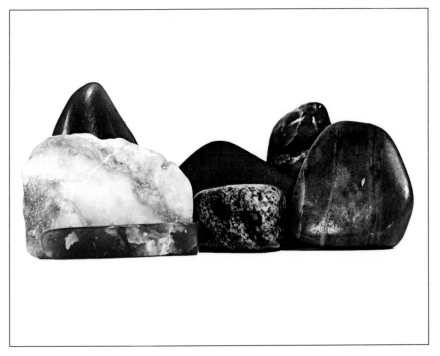

Jade from around the world

In times past, in the Far East and in the Americas, jade was revered more than any other precious substance. It is found on six out of the seven continents and occurs in a variety of colors. Although green is usually the most favored, jade may also be white, gray, brown, black, blue, yellow, orange, red, pink, and lavender. Jade is actually a family of two distinct metamorphic rocks: jadeite and nephrite. Nephrite jade is the commoner of the two, and it is the classical jade of China.

Jades are very durable gemstones, famous for withstanding the passage of time. Consequently, nearly every culture that had access to jade has associated it with health, longevity, and safe passage to the afterlife. Frequently, jade appears among votive offerings and funerary goods. Chinese emperors and the rulers of pre-Columbian cultures were buried with jade in order to ensure their entry into paradise.

Jade's primary effect is to instill peace. It works gently and gradually; its nature is not hurried at all. Peace is not an outer vibration that can be implanted. It is instead cultivated by letting go: letting go of anger, letting go of worry, letting go of attachment, and even letting go of time. Peace exists only in the present moment. Any emotion or attachment outside of the eternal Now counteracts the goal of peace. Jade is a timeless, eternal gemstone, one that encourages compassion and presence.

One function of jade is to embrace the inevitability of death. Our physical selves are ephemeral vehicles for an eternal spirit. Recognizing this simple truth supplants the efforts of the ego, which thrives on attachment, conflict, and fear. By continuously embracing jade's directive of awareness, one removes the mask of the ego that we wear and opens our eyes to a state of timelessness. By recognizing the true self, which exists beyond the earthly restrictions of time and space, we can see the influences of karma in our lives. Peaceful observance of how the law of cause and effect is coursing through our lives is often enough to release ourselves from the continuance of a karmic cycle.

Since jade is traditionally associated with ancient cultures and was sometimes handed down from generation to generation, it can also help to heal family karma.[21] It has a strong connection to the realm of the ancestors and to nonordinary reality or the dreamtime. Jade fosters an intimate link to other levels of reality in order to explore and release the karma held within these planes of existence. In doing so, we can apply jade to the amelioration of genealogical karma. It is a superb ally in shamanic journeying, too, and its presence can alert your guides and ancestors to your need for assistance in visiting past lives or releasing karmic ties.

Nephrite jade, in particular, focuses on embodiment of peace and compassion. In a very literal sense, the composition of jade resembles our connective tissue, which represents bringing forth peace from the most basic and fundamental aspect of our existence.[22] This enables us to generate merit through compassionate actions; it awakens the inner bodhisattva within each of us. Allowing jade into your life opens the doorway to good fortune, not because it attracts wealth or happiness, but because we generate good karma as we attune to its peaceful and loving energies.

KYANITE

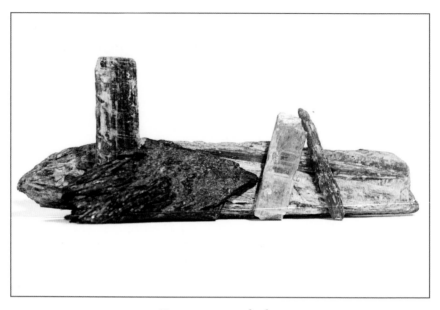

Kyanite in several colors

A silicate of aluminum, kyanite most often occurs as blue-bladed crystals in metamorphic rock. Kyanite is composed of thin crystalline layers laminated together to form a single crystal. Kyanite is strange in that it has two hardness values; one when tested along one axis and a different hardness when tested on another. It is a popular healing tool and is abundant in many collections today.

Blue kyanite is the most important for activating the causal chakra.[23] The causal plane is the connection between the highest dimensions and physical reality, and kyanite's role is to connect our lower selves to the causal plane. At the causal level we can see where the seeds of karma are sown into all experiences we manifest in life. Kyanite can align the conscious mind with the causal plane in order to bring a sense of calm and understanding while observing the karmic blueprints in action.

The domain of kyanite is primarily mental, and it therefore does not heal or release karma on its own. However, because it is so efficient at bridging the mental and causal planes, it can enable one to make a better connection to karmic patterns, both current and past, such that other karmic healing stones can eliminate and transmute their effects on our current life. It is an effective partner for any of the blueprint-healing stones such as diamond, aquamarine, and trigonic quartz. Kyanite supports an evolved level of consciousness; meditating with it opens the causal chakra. It can unite the higher spiritual parts of our beings with the lower self.

Black kyanite, unlike its blue siblings, forms as fan-shaped, radiating masses of tiny crystals. These kyanite fans can be used to rake or comb the causal body and other layers of the aura in order to remove karmic debris. Their specialized color diverts their energy away from the mental plane and into the karmic more than other forms of kyanite. Since their fundamental structure is unchanged, black kyanite crystals are excellent at facilitating connection; use them to traverse into the karmic, or causal, plane in order to enact lasting transformation.

Orange kyanite breathes new energy into a familiar stone. More recently available than other varieties of kyanite, this orange crystal stimulates better recall of memory, as well as a sense of timelessness. Like carnelian, it can help to build enough energy to break free from karmic patterns, but orange kyanite focuses this ability only at the mental level. Like other members of the kyanite clan, orange kyanite is an articulate bridge builder; it extends bridges not only from the mental to the causal bodies, but also from person to person. Orange kyanite promotes understanding of the karma extant in our relationships with one another. When more clarity is needed on this subject, use it in tandem with rhodochrosite in order to separate the emotional and mental debris that cloud understanding.

LAPIS LAZULI

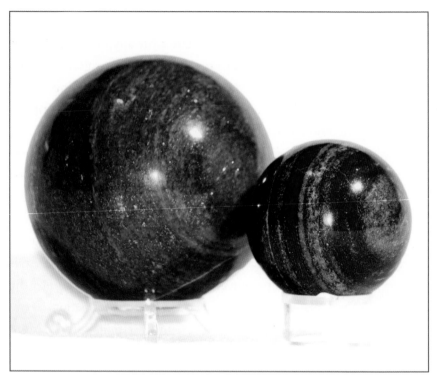

Lapis lazuli

Lapis lazuli is a metamorphic rock primarily composed of lazurite, calcite, and iron pyrite. Its color range goes from deep indigo to bright ultramarine, and it is often bedecked with white streaks and swirls as well as speckles of gold. Since antiquity this gemstone has been treasured for its celestial color and heavenly energy. It is a multifaceted healing tool, capable of working with both the heart and the mind, as well as helping ameliorate certain conditions in the physical body.

For karmic healing, lapis lazuli can be applied for overcoming negative karma through inspiring hope. This gem serves to enjoin the heart and the mind such that they work together toward a common goal. This eliminates inner conflict, which often gives rise to negative karma.

For this reason, lapis is a gentle healer that lifts away the negative experience of karma in order to focus more clearly on its deeper, often hidden causes.

Lapis is also a stone of the shaman's rebirth. In meditation, it helps to access the consciousness of the soul between lifetimes. In this in-between state, karma is both reviewed and meted out. Lapis can help to resolve karma by granting a fresh perspective on stale patterns. It helps disperse the indigo ray, which embodies the qualities associated with Saturn. As such, it can facilitate understanding of cause and effect, as well as offer both the intellectual and emotional understanding of the core structure of karmic patterns.

LEOPARDSKIN JASPER

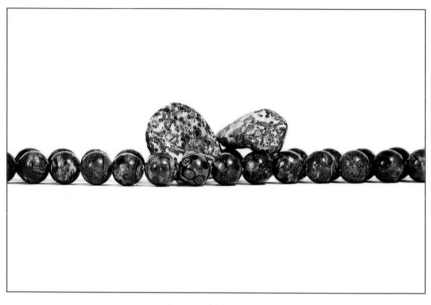

Leopardskin jasper

Leopardskin jasper, actually a form of rhyolite, is one of my favorite stones for karmic healing. Similar to true members of the jasper family, it is very grounding and stabilizing overall. The characteristic pattern, which resembles leopard spots, makes for a handsome gemstone or even a tumbled stone with personality.

As an igneous rock, leopardskin jasper promotes the understanding of our current situation as a result of the flux and crystallization of our causal realities. The karma we accumulate amalgamates into the reality we are currently experiencing. Leopardskin jaspar provides a down-to-earth approach to tackling karmic healing, and as a result it can be both catalyst and motivator. It fosters an earthy approach to viewing spiritual phenomena and helps to integrate the higher realities into the everyday. It is a lovely grounding stone, and it can help to counterbalance the effects of higher, more spiritually oriented gemstones and crystals.

Leopardskin jasper works to promote flexibility, centering, and understanding. Just as the spots appear on it in a repeating pattern, it helps to propagate the patterns for what we need in life within our aura. As these energetic seeds are repeated throughout our nonphysical bodies, we become seemingly magnetized to attract things into our life. An easygoing, trusting attitude is born out of this process, because it is easy to recognize that we are always supported.

Part of the reason that leopardskin jasper works so well to attract what we need is because it fine-tunes our sense of timing. The circular orbs from which it is composed act like knobs and dials to retune our experience of time and space. This strongly impacts the causal body, which processes the experience of time and memory. As we become better attuned to leopardskin jasper's regulatory function, we are more and more centered in the flow of infinite abundance within the universe, and perfect timing becomes second nature. The result of leopardskin jasper in causal healing is that one becomes more synchronized with the timing of the planet, the flow of the universe, and the rhythms expressed in one's blueprint.

The longer you wear or carry this stone, the more profound its effect. Essentially, it continues to "clear, adjust, and harmonize all the clockwork type mechanisms that regulate and govern all body processes."[24] This tends to saturate the physical body first, and then move outward. As one becomes better attuned to leopardskin jasper, you find that everything in life just seems to work out better than ever. Truthfully, what is happening is that you are more aligned to the rhythm of the universe and to your karmic blueprint, so that there is less opportunity for friction in life.

OBSIDIAN

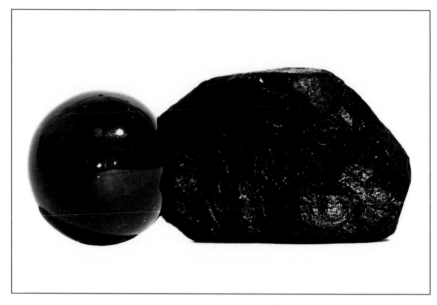

Obsidian, raw and polished

Obsidian is a natural glass, traditionally formed as silica-rich lava cools rapidly. Since it hardens so quickly, crystals are unable to form; the end result is a vitreous, amorphous rock. Long-praised for its sharpness and reflective qualities, obsidian is a natural stone for karmic support. It is grounding, protective, and insightful, and it can be a wonderful ally in many avenues of healing.

Obsidian spheres and mirrors make for excellent scrying tools. They may be directed to grant visions of past or future lives, and they may also be queried for insight into the origin of a specific pattern or cycle of karma that recurs in your life. Tumbled obsidian can also be placed on the third eye to help confront the shadow aspects of our lives, such as those responsible for the negative karma we have generated. Obsidian is sometimes a ruthless teacher, so caution and patience are recommended when working in this way.

As a dark, noncrystalline tool, obsidian helps us look at the darkness in order to bring it into the light. Obsidian can overcome the fear of karma itself or the antecedent in a long chain of karmic events in our lives. It helps us confront these fears and cut through the illusions surrounding them. This will bring us into a state of nonattachment and nonjudgment. In this space we are able to effectively handle the needs of our karma, either through release, integration, or learning a lesson that keeps coming up.

Many native cultures used obsidian in producing tools with sharp cutting edges, such as knives, spear points, and arrowheads. It is a sharp stone with equally sharp spiritual effects. It cuts through the illusion that we are our stories. No one is reduced to being only the results of karma; rather, karma tells the story of where we have been and how we got to where we are today. Karma does not tell us who we are, only what we have done. In this way obsidian offers strength, self-confidence, and the determination necessary to cut karmic ties and break away from repeating patterns in our lives.

Thanks to its amorphous structure, obsidian represents the cosmic void out of which manifest reality is birthed. Our spiritual templates are created from the same void, and this stone can initiate contact with the void. In this way we can experience the raw potential for creating or re-creating anything and everything. In this state, it is easier to heal or adjust our blueprint and to rewrite soul contracts, too.

OPAL

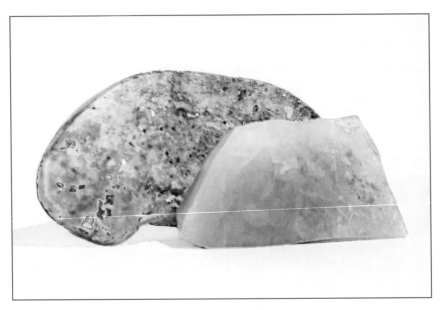

Australian opal

Opals are an amorphous silica famous for an iridescent or opalescent play of colors. While not all opals exhibit this phenomenon, all opals are made of spheres of silica stacked together with water molecules interspersed among them. When the silica globes are of relatively similar size and are stacked in regular patterns, and when the water is evenly distributed, the end result is a beautiful, flashy opal. Opals are found in various parts of the world, with nongem-quality specimens available in many colors, both translucent and opaque.

Opal has an amplifying effect like its silica-based cousin, quartz, although its energy is much more diffuse. Precious opals are versatile healers because of the extraordinarily diverse number of colors within them. The water content of all opals attunes their energy to the realm of the subconscious mind and to the emotions. The mystical play of color and light in many opals initiates connection to cosmic states of consciousness.[25] Opals are visionary gemstones, and they can accordingly enhance spiritual sight by sharpening the intuition and heightening visionary experiences.

Since opals are often formed by sedimentary activity, they direct their light into the past. They are especially effective for cultivating wisdom predicated on the experience of past lives and our past decisions in this life. Opals also reveal what is beneath our emotional state by allowing previous influences on the emotions to come to light. Furthermore, they engender a sense of responsibility, thereby encouraging you to act on this knowledge. This, in turn, can allow you to take control of your emotions and to reverse the karmic effects of your past decisions.

Being an amorphous gemstone, opals lack any true crystalline structure. This lack of crystallinity represents the premanifest state, sometimes referred to as the cosmic void. It is in this void that our soul incubates between incarnations on the Earth plane. The void is a cauldron of transformation and the womb of potential. Just like the mother's womb, opals are aqueous stones; they take us back into the void of becoming in order to instill a primordial sense of innocence. Through this return to innocence, opals initiate a state of complete and utter surrender to grace. The frequency of grace is the remedy for all negative karma, for it allows for atonement and healing. When we connect to opals on the most primal level, they wash over us with this grace, and we are set free from the ties that bind us. We are returned to unimaginable possibility.

Banded Opal and Boulder Opal

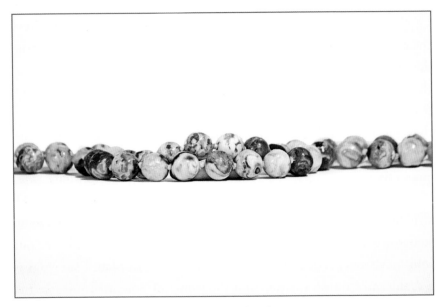

Banded opal beads

Banded opal and boulder opal are two different members of the opal family with similar missions. Banded opal is sometimes called *opalite;* it is a nonprecious, milky opal in its host matrix. When polished, the sedimentary layers of opal and host rock are revealed in a banded pattern. Boulder opal is another opal in its host matrix, although it typically refers to flashes of precious opal in a dark matrix stone. Occasionally, this opal formation also occurs in banded layers or concentric patterns. These matrix opals are held within their mother rock. They emphasize the motherly aspect of opal, in which our causal existence is wrapped up in a virtual hug. They can help us to be more objective about our karma, since they soothe away any emotional rawness from our current experiences. Their structure is much denser than precious opals, and that provides a grounding element to their energy, too.

Banded opal is especially effective for resolving karma. Its mission is to sift through the causal aura, or the memory body, and to highlight the areas of karma active in our lives.[26] The opal is formed by sedimentary processes, giving it a particular affinity with time and karma. Just as our current scenario in life is the result of all of our previous decisions and actions, sedimentary rocks form from the buildup of minute rock particles. These crystallize together over the eons to produce new rocks. Matrix opals, both banded and boulder varieties, form from sedimentary action, and they offer their own expertise with time.

The causal body is most active when we sleep because the dreamtime is an excellent vehicle for the mind to review and process karma. Many dreams are products of this review process, which is why unexpected memories can feature into dreams. The mind is sorting through the causal body trying to extricate karma from the present moment through the dream state. Oftentimes we are unable or unwilling to fully release our ties to the past. This is where opal comes into play. Opals can be worn to bed or placed under the pillow to assist in the unconscious release of karma.

Opals in their matrix assist the higher mind to see the karmic roots of any condition, and they can improve your chances of releasing karma. They identify the areas in greatest need of karmic resolution and offer a gently grounding force, thus providing an outlet to release any emotional attachment maintaining the karmic energy so that it may be relinquished to and transmuted by the Earth. Next, opal allows the meaning or lesson of one's karma to be fully integrated prior to release. In the final stage, opal helps to sever the link to the past by infusing the area with light and positivity; even opals without the gemmy opalescence have this luminous capacity.

Green Opal

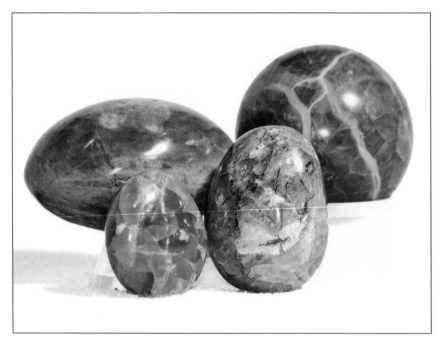

Green opal from Madagascar

Green opal is strongly centered at the physical level. Its energy gently flows into the body and offers rejuvenation to our weakest organs and tissues. Green opal aids the immune system and the heart; it's a great go-to gemstone for colds, flu, and sinus issues, too.[27] The energy of this opal is brimming with youthfulness, joy, and freshness. It can help stagnant cycles in our lives finally take a step into a new direction.

Green opals rarely have the fiery play of color present in more precious varieties of opal. Because of this, they shift their focus to understanding karmic patterns rather than releasing them. When repeated illness or conditions affect the physical body, green opal can offer insight into the karmic background of these disorders. It is a gentle reminder that our higher mind is a powerful tool for shaping our experience of the physical world, including the lessons of karma.

Green opal gives meaning to everyday life by granting a more spiritual perspective to the material plane. It serves as a welcome teacher, revealing and reminding us that the material world is the classroom of the soul, therefore each challenge we face is really an opportunity to integrate a new lesson. When we choose to embrace the friction in our lives as a learning opportunity, we tend to generate more good karma than bad, and we can foster an understanding of the weight of the karma we have brought into this plane from previous lifetimes, too. It is an excellent mental and emotional filter, engendering a more inno-cent state of mind to the spiritual aspirant, and it makes every day a little more joyful. Green opal works to offer a sense of gratitude in the face of each karmic pattern, and the wellspring of gratitude rising up from within can surmount any obstacle.

Pink Opal

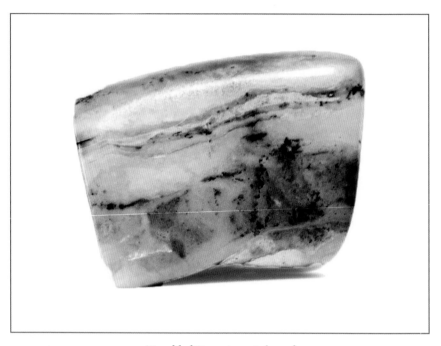

Tumbled Peruvian pink opal

Pink opal is usually opaque to subtranslucent, and it is often found in the Andes Mountains in Peru. It brings the state of grace to the heart center, grace being the highest and best equalizer of karmic debts. When meditating with or wearing pink opal it can also reveal the causal patterns that motivate the emotional body. In our auras, the emotional and causal bodies often work together. Much like rhodochrosite's action of supporting the release of causal energy from the emotional body, pink opal can separate emotional patterns from the causal body. By unwinding the confused energy patterns in our auras, healthy function can be restored or replenished even without release of emotions or karma. Pink opal is soothing, soft, and hopeful. It teaches that through grace and compassion, wholeness is available to us exactly where we are.

Welo Opal

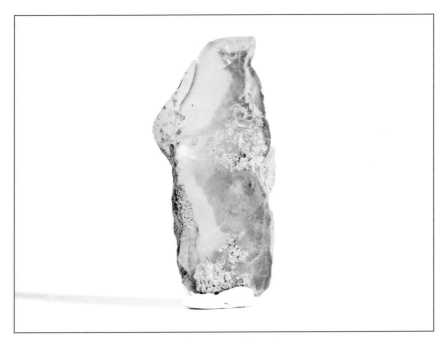

Ethiopian Welo opal

Welo opal is a precious opal recently discovered in Ethiopia, in Wollo Province, from which it derives its name. This opal, also called "Ethiopian opal" and "crystal opal" for its striking clarity, is one of the most enchanting members of the opal family. It is found in a variety of colors, and most specimens exhibit at least some of the opalescent fire for which opal is best known. The finest of these opals are clear enough to be faceted and still share their mystic play of color within the stone.

These newcomers to the opal clan offer a new octave of opal energy to the world. Welo opals convey a greater sense of crystalline light than any of the other opals. Their energy is much more intense and more spiritually focused. One of the primary functions of this opal is to burn away karma.[28] They are guides and teachers on the path of evolution, since they have undergone their own evolution.

Ethiopian opals are joyful stones, and they activate and unify the crown, heart, and base chakras.[29] They are also effective protection stones. Rather than erecting a barrier around your energy field to deflect unwanted frequencies, Welo opal fortifies your own connection to divine light. This neutralizes negative and disharmonious vibrations altogether, for your benefit and for the benefit of those around you. When consciously focused on the causal body, the same effect applies toward taking on negative karma; the light of Welo opal overpowers the amplitude of the karmic field, thus carrying it into a sympathetic vibration.

Ethioipian opals are some of the most potent tools for releasing karma. Their crystalline clarity and fiery brilliance work to incinerate our karma. Combining these gems with spirit quartz can direct this karmic release outward and onto a global scale. They may prove to be important tools for the evolution of the planet at this pivotal time in history.

PERIDOT

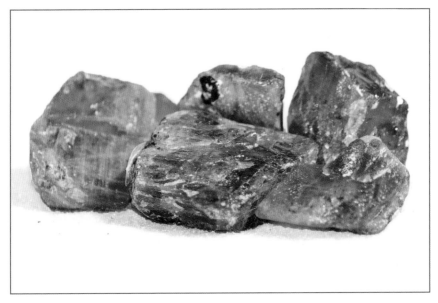

Crystals of peridot

Manganese-rich olivine is typically referred to as *peridot* in its gem-quality form. Its color, influenced by its iron content, is olive green. Peridot forms in igneous rocks, especially those rich in iron and manganese. While olivine crystals are common in mafic lavas and xenoliths, gemmy peridot accounts for only a small fraction. Rarely, peridot is found suspended in the nickel-iron matrix of pallasite meteorites.

Ancient sources point toward protective influences when peridot is worn; it is said to be a stone of overall health, wealth, and protection. It is also thought to confer spiritual growth, and it especially helps to reconcile relationships with money in many ways. Peridot can be considered a stone of spiritual wealth, and its action helps to release the underlying beliefs and karma of money. Meditating with or wearing this green crystal can help undo the momentum of karmic patterns of poverty and scarcity. It can help release ingrained beliefs around money carried over from previous lifetimes, as well as soften the effects of learned behaviors and ideas about money from earlier in your current lifetime. Peridot has a detoxifying effect on the physical body, and when applied toward the karma of money it is similarly effective in purging limiting cycles of poverty consciousness. Peridot can shake up the clauses in your soul contract governing your habits of spending and saving, and it can empower you to make better financial decisions.

To best harness the energy of peridot for karmic healing, try meditating with a piece at the solar plexus. As you breathe, visualize its energy reaching through the core of your being as it seeks out outdated causal patterns. Peridot has a refreshing, rejuvenating effect. Working with it can bring hope where there was once despair, and it encourages shrewd, safe financial decisions. Use it in tandem with green apophyllite in order to deepen the reach of releasing causal energy related to money and wealth.

PIETERSITE

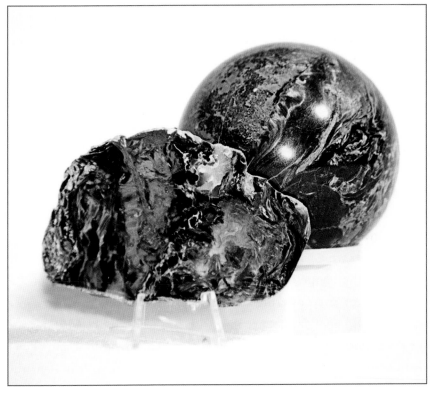

Namibian pietersite

Pietersite, also known as "tempest stone," is another quartz gemstone, and it is closely related to tiger's eye. Pietersite forms as quartz replaces fibers of asbestos-like minerals in the mineral formation riebeckite. The beautiful and velvety chatoyancy in this gemstone is attributed to the fibrous quality of its composition. Unlike tiger's eye, pietersite's patterns are bent and broken. They are swirled together in an almost chaotic, stormy mass. The colors in which this gemstone are found include golden, red, brown, blue, gray, green, and hints of purple. Although originally discovered in Namibia, a similar material was briefly available from China, with only a nominal difference in composition. Today pietersite is quite scarce.

Pietersite shares many characteristics with its cousins in the tiger's eye family. For example, it is grounding and can lend a supportive hand when you feel out of balance. Unlike other stones, though, pietersite grounds your consciousness to the etheric body rather than the earth; this enables astral travel and shamanic journeying, as well as past-life exploration. Pietersite is sometimes called "eagle's eye," which implies its aptitude in offering a better perspective on the situations we experience in our current lives or in past-life regressions.

The stormy appearance of pietersite points toward its greatest strength: it churns the energy of your subtle body, loosening the grip of emotional trauma. It teaches you to weather the storms in life, and it can be especially helpful to those who connect intimately to storm energy and symbolism. When life appears to be in chaos, such as when the tides of karma have swept us up, pietersite comes in to act as a life preserver. The tempest stone specializes in transformation. It can feel destructive or overpowering at first, but thereafter it leaves you in a refreshed and energized state. Pietersite is a powerful cleansing stone for the aura. It unravels the energies that are stuck within it and allows them to be sorted by the appropriate layer of the aura. It loosens the grip of karma in your causal body, thereby allowing you to store the memory of the event in the causal body without the negative side effects of its karmic action.

Pietersite also awakens our cells during the transformational processes, helping them to process and purge any causal information stored in the DNA that is no longer supportive of your evolutionary direction. As you continue to evolve, the tempest stone teaches "how to align with the divine ideal."[30] Furthermore, as it guides in aligning with the blueprint, pietersite enables you to feel more comfortable and supported throughout the process. Ultimately, it reminds you that you are "an unlimited, divine, creative being within the structure of the Cosmic Plan."[31]

Like tiger's eye, pietersite is closely linked to power and the will. It helps you to claim your personal power and access the right use of the will, such as was shut down after the end of Atlantis. Pietersite teaches you to bring your passion, soul, and perseverance into your spiritual work, or any other work for that matter, in order to allow you to more fully live and walk your truth. When we become more fully aligned to our sense of truth, we can walk safely on the path to our destiny.

PRESELI BLUESTONE

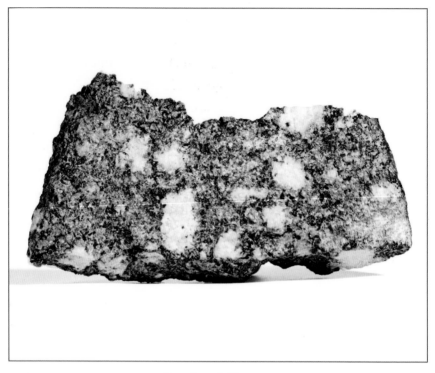

Raw Preseli bluestone

Eons ago, large pieces of bluestone, a variety of dolerite, were transported from Wales to the Salisbury Plain during the construction of Stonehenge. This igneous rock, the same stone that the ancient stone monoliths at Stonehenge are made from, is a mixture of various minerals, including plagioclase feldspar, augite, and olivine, with trace amounts of copper, magnetite, quartz, apatite, calcite, hornblende, and various other rock-forming minerals.[32] It is a grayish, blue-green color, with patches of lighter and darker minerals. Bluestone often slowly transforms from greenish or bluish to reddish over time as it is exposed to the elements.

This rock conveys a sense of timelessness and wisdom when held. Preseli bluestone, named for a range of hills in North Pembrokeshire,

West Wales, feels ancient and all-knowing, as if it has witnessed all of history. Connecting to its energy opens a doorway to the record of Earth's past and future changes. It is deeply in tune with the passage of the seasons and the rhythms of the stars. Preseli bluestone supports and nourishes the earth star chakra, which enables it to serve as an anchor during shamanic journeys and astral travel.

Preseli bluestone is helpful in guiding the consciousness backward in time. It can be used to facilitate past-life exploration and for shifting the karmic imprints left by the actions of our previous incarnations. The impact of bluestone in one's energy field is at once protective and expansive, thereby allowing the sense of self to "expand beyond the normal experience of time and space."[33] As this healing stone is used to explore concurrent lifetimes, it can shed light on otherwise unknown or hidden patterns; it especially "helps the recognition of repeating, but hidden, patterns of perception and behaviour."[34]

Working with Preseli bluestone is not limited to exploring and releasing personal karma. This stone is attuned to the energies of Earth as a planetary whole, and it facilitates karmic release on the family, community, national, and global levels. It is a helpful adjunct to other stones for karmic release because its energy is so stabilizing; it can counter the emotional release that often accompanies realization and release of causal patterns. Bluestone is an insightful teacher and tool; it sharpens the memories of past lives, aids shamanic journeys, and emphasizes the interconnectedness of all life forms, objects, and places on planet Earth.

QUARTZ

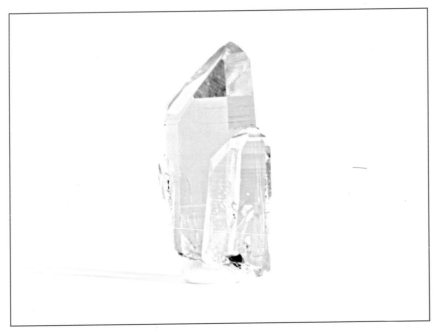

Clear quartz

A staple of all collections, quartz is easily the most recognizable and the most universally applicable gemstone in the healing arts. It is found all over the world, in more colors, shapes, and configurations than are imaginable. Quartz is the ideal all-purpose stone, and it offers healing benefits at virtually every level of one's being. Although most quartz is not specifically geared to karmic healing, specific varieties with causal influences are outlined in the pages that follow.*

---

*The terms *Dow, elestial, record keeper, laser wand,* and *time link* were first described in Katrina Raphaell's Crystal Trilogy: *Crystal Enlightenment, Crystal Healing,* and *The Crystalline Transmission.*

Dow Crystal

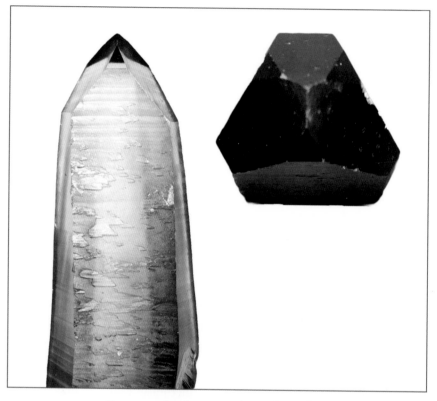

Dow crystal, side view and view from above

One of the most potent tools of transformation, the Dow crystal exhibits geometrical perfection among the arrangement of its termination faces. These special quartz crystals have points composed of alternating triangles and heptagons; this pattern appears to form a mandala when viewed from the end of the crystal. The Dow crystal is named for JaneAnn Dow, whose work with them and exploration into their numerology provided the very first insight into the capacity of these crystals.

The Dow crystal is considered to be one of the twelve "master crystals," a group of twelve special formations of quartz first described by noted crystal healer and author Katrina Raphaell. These formations of quartz are the crystalline masters and teachers for the evolution of consciousness on the planet. The Dow is actually a combination of two of the other master crystals: the transmitter and the channeling crystals.[35] In addition to being fine tools of transmitting and receiving messages from the nonphysical planes, the Dow crystal also expresses a perfected, crystalline order. This is apparent in its beautifully arranged terminal facets. These geometric faces represent the attainment of perfection, truth, and co-creating positive change. As such it is a template for accessing and attaining Christ consciousness. Because of its innate perfection, the Dow teaches that we are able to "physically manifest [the same] state of integrity, unity, balance and order."[36] These crystals bring us into deeper awareness of our blueprint, and they represent this shift through the trinity of their design. The triangles in their apexes "represent the body, mind, and spirit balance so necessary for us to reach our spiritual perfection."[37]

Those who are attracted to Dows may be experiencing a conflict between their spiritual blueprint and their current scenario.[38] The Dow crystal, with its idealized morphology, resonates at a frequency that highlights this dissonance and brings it to a head in order to be reviewed. It is excellent when used in meditation, and it may also be placed on the body during healing for this purpose. Connecting to the energy of this crystal will "emphasize the perfection innate in all of our patterning, rather than actualizing it."[39] In other words, the Dow's mission is not to correct the expression of your blueprint; instead it allows you to understand when you are in conflict with your blueprint.

Because of its ability to instill recognition of the information in the blueprint, the Dow crystal partners well with diamond, aquamarine, and trigonic crystal. It shines a bright light into the discordant areas of life that are not in harmony with the blueprint. These other crystals can also help to usher the inherent perfection of the blueprint into these zones of disharmony. Shungite as well can be used with the Dow in order to cleanse information that conflicts with the patterning of the soul.

Elestial Crystal

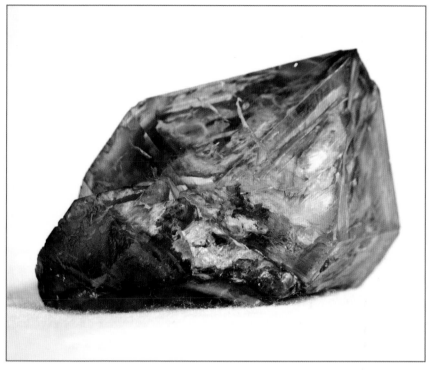

A smoky elestial

The elestial is less well-defined than other quartz morphologies. Unlike other formations, the geological mechanisms for creating elestials are varied. Their intriguing patterns result from a variety of mineralogical processes such as parallel growth, sceptered crystals, skeletal growth, and twinning. Terminations and hollow etchings may cascade all along the surfaces of elestial quartz. The overall appearance resembles a geometrical encoding. Elestials are defined as much by their energy as they are by their appearance. Most elestials occur as smoky quartz, although they are also found in other varieties of quartz, including amethyst, rose quartz, clear quartz, and citrine.

Elestial crystals are masters of releasing trapped emotions. The striking geometries of elestials render them capable of resonating with our own encoding. They work predominantly at the emotional body, helping to loosen the hold of outdated patterns. Elestials can also be applied to other layers of the aura and to each of the chakras with similar results. Due to their special morphology, elestial crystals help to restructure energy fields.[40] They can be used to purify the nonphysical anatomy by releasing the causal energies embedded within them.

Working like repositories of information, each crystallized growth on the elestial is like a different book in a library. They are storehouses of sacred information relevant to the progression of the soul. Elestial crystals help to adjust and inform our life choices in accordance with understanding from a more spiritually advanced perspective. Elestials feel like wise old beings, and they may help in providing insight into patterns established in previous lifetimes.

Smoky elestials are the most fortifying of the elestial family. They serve to stabilize and anchor the consciousness through the evolving energies of the current changes. Working with these crystals is a sacred experience; they seem to grow with you in a way that one never outgrows. They may be applied to the solar plexus to release stored memories of pain, including karmic impressions contained there. Like all elestials, they help to heal at the soul level, often by supplying additional reinforcement to our structural integrity; this function allows them to serve as stepping-stones to better expressing our spiritual blueprint.

Smoky elestials appear as if they have been created by a confluence of the four alchemical elements.[41] Their multiple terminations often appear singed, and their heft underpins their earthy characteristics. Quartz often forms from an aqueous solution, and the elestials retain a touch of that watery nature. Additionally, the clarity often hidden in their cores is reminiscent of the clear, airy cavities and caves in which they are sometimes found. In this way, elestial crystals help to supply all the tools necessary for evolution and alchemy. They are stones of transition, never failing to provide the catalyst needed for spiritual unfoldment.

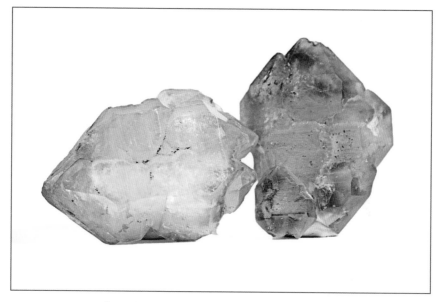

Amethyst elestials from Kenya and from North Carolina

Amethyst elestials are unique and complex crystals. In addition to the abilities of amethyst described previously, these crystals exhibit the effects of amethyst, too. Since amethyst elestials focus the energy into the spiritual bodies, they can act as tools for purging causal information and attachments from the other bodies. Amethystine elestial quartz feels as though it is rewriting the encoded information of the spiritual self. This makes it an apt tool for rewriting one's soul contract by purging any agreements that no longer encourage growth and wholeness. Amethyst itself works to release limiting beliefs and energies, so the pairing of the purple amethyst with the geometric energy of elestials enables them to encourage release at the karmic level. These sacred crystals can permit long-lasting changes to be made that allow you to move in new directions, away from the cycles of pain or disharmony you may have experienced.

Glacial Etched Quartz

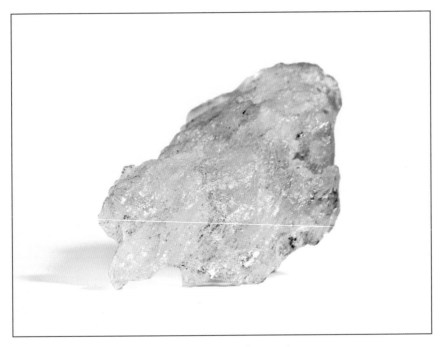

Glacial etched quartz from Pakistan

Glacial etched quartz represents a family of quartz crystals found in the Himalayas and nearby locations. All of the crystals exhibit a form of surface etching or growth interference caused by special circumstances in their formation environments. Many have unusual patterns and markings etched on their surfaces. The most famous of these crystals come from Kullu Pass, India, and they are variously known as Kullu rosies, Himalayan ice quartz, and nirvana quartz. Other forms of glacial etched quartz may be found in Pakistan and Nepal, and they may be accompanied by interesting inclusions of a variety of minerals.

Much glacial quartz has been found as glaciers recede; these strange crystals found beneath the cover of the glaciers often resemble the icy glaciers themselves. It has been postulated that the deglaciation of the region may be a reflection of global warming and the overall transition occurring on Earth. The crystals of this area have always seemed to reflect a level of reassurance about these Earth changes. Although the actions of humankind may be accelerating these changes (and accruing the associated karma for doing so), the glacial etched crystals remind us that it is all a part of the divine plan. This can help to redirect the causal energy of Earth changes, such as global warming, and focus it on learning patterns rather than as reaping the effects of negative karma. These crystals also help eliminate a sense of victimhood at the karmic level; the end result is instead empowering, and it allows you to take control of your life.

The glacial etched crystals from India, such as the nirvana quartz, display growth interference from calcite crystals once having grown around the quartz. These calcites are later swept away, leaving only the more stable quartz in place. This results in striking and unconventional crystals that teach us to look at the cause of a specific condition or cycle. Just like the quartz crystals exhibiting what would be otherwise impossible geometry, the current condition may seem to be out of its karmic or causal context. These sacred forms of quartz release you from your karmically driven relationship cycles; they enable you to cease the

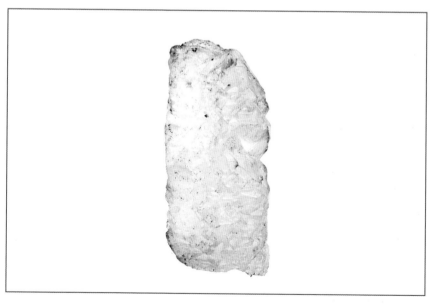

Nirvana quartz, also called Himalayan ice quartz

pattern as you gather perspective into what you are repeating time and time again.

Glacial etched crystals, especially the variety from the Kullu Pass, are also predisposed to displaying trigonic markings. This endows them with all of the properties of trigonic crystals, which are described on page 162. They are dynamic and powerful soul-level healers, and they can help access and align our blueprint information.

Lemurian Seed Crystals

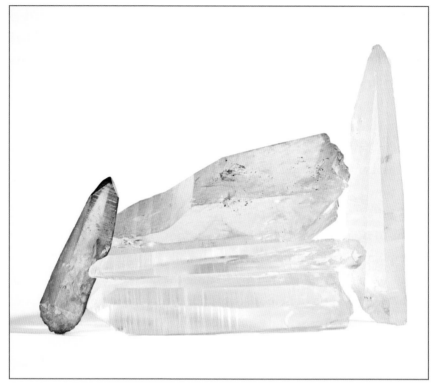

Lemurian seed crystals

Lemurian seed crystals are traditionally found in Serra do Cabral, Brazil, although nowadays several locations across the planet produce Lemurian crystals. Most are configured as laser wands and are excellent tools for energy healing. They are recognized by a distinctive Muzo habit, in which the crystals have a triangular or nearly triangular cross section and pronounced horizontal striations on the widest faces of the body of the crystal. They were first discovered in Brazil in the year 2000, and Katrina Raphaell was the first writer to report their energies.

The seed crystals are named for the continent of Lemuria, an ancient land now lost beneath the Pacific Ocean. Lemurian society was spiritually very advanced, not unlike Atlantis. However, this manifested as a more intuitive, feminine way of life, more in tune with nature than that of the Atlanteans. Lemuria is sometimes viewed as the original birthplace of humankind, much like the Garden of Eden, and researchers have attributed its loss to a variety of different causes. No matter how it sank, the disappearance of Lemuria presaged a time in which humanity would lose the balance and harmony typified by Lemurian consciousness. Before their disappearance, select members of Lemurian society encoded the wisdom and memory of their ways into the Lemurian seed crystals to be rediscovered by humanity at the right time.

Similar to record keeper crystals, Lemurian seed crystals are meant to be repositories of ancient wisdom. They are located in strategic points worldwide in order to broadcast their frequencies into the surrounding quartz, thereby seeding the crystals with the wisdom of ancient Lemuria. The horizontal lines emblazoned on the sides of these special quartz crystals are Lemurian record keepers in their own right.

Lemurian seed crystals can be used to access past-life information, especially as related to the lost civilization of Lemuria. Place the striations against the third eye in meditation to accomplish this. These crystals can also facilitate travel to Lemurian past lives in order to clarify why these lifetimes are influencing a person's karma. It may be necessary to combine them with a stone better suited to journeying to better achieve this outcome. Some relatives of these crystals, such as the Lemurian dreamtime phantoms from Australia, are geared to shamanic journeying. Some newer Brazilian Lemurian seed crystals also exhibit beautiful phantoms, thereby equipping them for past-life journeys.

When working with a Lemurian seed crystal for karmic healing, its wand-like shape enables it to cut karmic cords and to encapsulate karmic patterns in the aura for removal and release. These crystals make deft energy scalpels for all sorts of energetic healing applications.

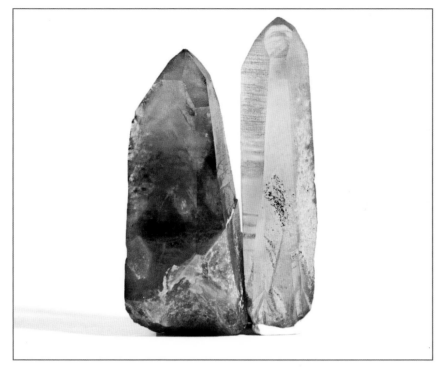

Lemurian dreamtime phantom crystal (left)
and green phantom Lemurian seed crystal (right)

They emanate an energy of peace, love, and oneness, which translates to remediating the effects of negative karma. Placing one on the heart after removing or resolving a particular karmic pattern may facilitate more lasting results.

Lemurian seed crystals offer the ability to reprogram our karmic bodies through the etched lines along their sides. Sweeping them through the aura can help to replace old karmic patterns with a specific intention. They can also remove karmic debris when moved through the causal body and the etheric body, and Lemurian crystals may thereby help to rewrite your soul imperatives. This enables you to end a pattern or cycle even before the karmic lesson has finished playing out, in order to move into a healthier and more joyful direction.

The Lemurian seeds are also beautiful additions to any grids for releasing karma on a global level, as they work to reestablish the patterns of energy that existed prior to Atlantis. The Lemurian culture exhibited behavior and intention on the opposite side of the spectrum from that of Atlantis; they were much more in tune with their spiritual place in the universe. In this way, Lemurian seed crystals may offer balance to the negative karma Earth as a whole experienced during the destruction of Atlantis.

Phantom Crystal

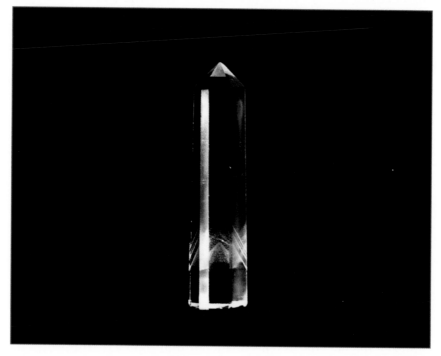

Phantoms in quartz

Phantom crystals have an image of their former selves frozen within them. Usually phantoms occur as changes in the formation environment interrupt or slow the growth of a crystal. In many instances another mineral may be added to the mix, such as hematite or chlorite, resulting in a colored phantom highlighted by the accessory mineral. Phantom crystals are not limited to quartz, and they are often found in selenite, calcite, and fluorite, and many more minerals.

Phantom quartz is the ultimate past-life crystal. Changes made to the crystal during earlier phases of its growth are recorded within the body of the stone. This represents the effects of our past and future lives during the evolution of the soul. These crystals exhibit the stages of development of their previous selves in a manner that facilitates past-life regression. When the soul repeats the same pattern in multiple lives, it is often because a karmic lesson has not been learned. Phantom quartz guides the user to the first instance in which such a causal cycle began. Doing so may enable one to learn and integrate this lesson completely in the current lifetime.

When phantom crystals are formed, their growth may appear to start and stop many times. Indeed, some crystals display dozens and dozens of phantoms upon close inspection. At no point did the crystal give up its quest to form merely because a new challenge or deviation came into play; it instead grew around the obstacle, encapsulating that moment as a ghostly impression of its former morphology. The lesson these crystals teach through this is that karmic lessons are meant to be integrated rather than pushed away. We grow with them as we internalize their opportunities, rather than try to avoid them for fear that they are hindrances. Phantom crystals actually propel us on our path despite karmic limitations.

Phantom crystals may facilitate access to the Akashic records in meditation. Additionally, they allow insight into the prebirth state and stimulate the impetus to renegotiate our soul contracts. This works by reframing the context of our past lives, as well as the memories of our current life, in a way that celebrates the lessons without handing our awareness over to pain. They are competent healers of the shadow self and may be used in a multitude of healing scenarios

Record Keepers

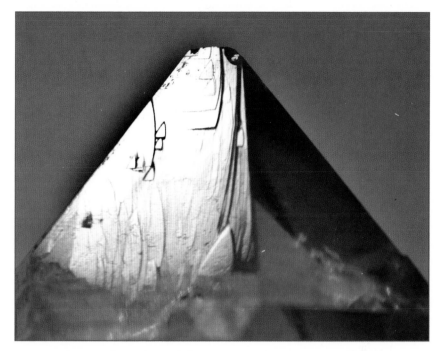

Close-up of record-keeper formations on the termination of quartz

Record keeper crystals are identified by upward-pointing triangles raised or etched onto the faces of a crystal point.[42] Sometimes these patterns are etched so faintly that they are difficult to find, and it is necessary to pay close attention in order to locate them. Record keepers are believed to contain specific information programmed within them, typically meant for a certain person. When you find one of these special quartzes, you may discover a virtual treasure trove of information within it during meditation.

The record keepers are thought to have originated in Atlantis. Since the Atlantean society was so in tune with crystal energy, they were able to co-creatively grow unique formations of quartz and other minerals to meet their exact needs. The birth of the triangular markings represented a modified way of storing information. It became possible for people to store memories and instructions in the record keepers for future use. Over time, this became imperative as a means of saving a record of Atlantean teachings for a time when humanity would be ready.

The purpose of record keeper crystals was first discovered in the 1980s. When this information was made available, they were relatively uncommon crystal formations. As the collective consciousness of the planet has healed and transformed, more record keepers have been made available. There are even instances of spontaneous appearances of these markings on the surface of crystals once they have come in contact with the person they are meant to be with.

Record keepers have been programmed such that they will awaken in the hands of their caretakers when approached with an open and sincere heart.[43] The information within them may have been placed there by your own soul during a previous lifetime. Some of these stones have actually been seeded by higher beings to prepare the planet for our current phase of evolution. Holding a record keeper can often feel like coming home, and for this reason they often become personal sacred meditation tools.

To work with a record keeper, place the face with the triangular markings against the heart or the third eye. Conversely, you can meditate by gazing at or into the triangles themselves. In meditation, one may be granted access to the past-life wisdom kept within these sacred crystals. Flashes of insight, scenes from past lives, and even information relevant to your current life can be found there. By journeying into the crystals during meditation, some record keepers will give you access to the Akashic records themselves. It is worth experimenting to see if they do!

Record keepers generally are teaching crystals. They do not initiate the healing of karma on their own, although the insight they provide may allow their caretakers to make a conscious decision to release and overcome karmic influences. To carry the effects of record keepers into the realm of healing, try combining them with stones such as

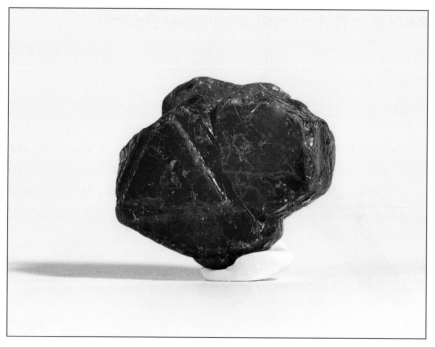

Record keeper on ruby

Ethiopian opal or banded opal. These gems will help to resolve and burn away the karmic influence of the past-life information unveiled by the record keeper.

Although typically discussed only in their form as quartz, record keeper crystals may occur in other mineral forms, too. In such instances they offer a combination of the above information with the general qualities of the host mineral. Examples of other record keepers include corundum (ruby and sapphire), diamond, and calcite. Examine your crystal tool kit and you may discover a record keeper among your treasures.

Red Laser Quartz and Amphibole Quartz

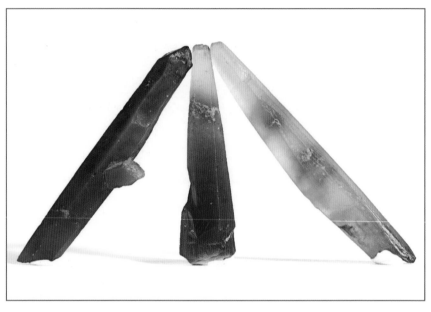

Laser wands colored by amphibole and hematite

Red laser quartz describes a form of amphibole-included crystal whose red color is owed to tinges of hematite. These crystals have a tapering crystal habit ending in minute termination faces; the overall form of laser crystals is that of a wand or precision tool. Their exact color is more of an orangey red, and many exhibit clear portions, too. Similar crystals may be found in Brazil, China, and Madagascar. Their inclusions may resemble phantoms, and in these cases the properties of phantom crystals also apply. Other forms of amphibole quartz have similar qualities, and they are included here accordingly.

Red quartz is simultaneously grounding and energizing, largely due to its iron component. The warm, vital color of these crystals belies a fiery quality to their mission. They can be used to direct purifying flames into the causal body in order to burn away the karma stored there. Their dual appearance of being both reddish and clear has a regulatory function in that they moderate the inflow and outflow of causal information among each layer of the aura. Like the fibrous morphology of the amphibole within these red crystals, our causal bodies are often teeming with karmic ties and cords. Red laser quartz can encapsulate these energies in order to help remove them without depleting your energy.

The sharp, tapering morphology of these laser wands lends itself to cutting cords and performing auric surgery. Their inner fire offers a self-cauterizing feature, sealing the aura and safeguarding against recurring conditions. These crystals can best be applied to energy cords that have a karmic origin; in many cases they will be anchored in the causal body itself, though this is not a rule. Use the points as scalpels to cut through the cords, and reverse them to seal the aura with the crystals' bases. Similarly, the terminations can be directed at a blockage or stagnant area in any chakra to help instigate movement.

Amphibole, one of the constituents of this crystal's inner landscape, is often associated with angelic energy. Amphibole in quartz makes the

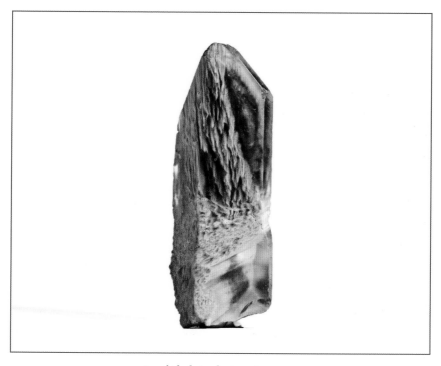

Amphibole inclusions in quartz

presence of angels in our lives more tangible. It gently attunes our frequency to that of the angels, which allows us to be better servants of God. Since many of these red wands are also singing crystals—that is, they produce a ringing or tinkling sound when struck gently—they help us hear the whispers of the divine all around us. They are sacred tools for reminding us that we are always supported on our journey to wholeness, especially when we seek to release the ties of karma in our lives.

Amphibole in quartz, more generally speaking, has the effect of aligning and fine-tuning the individual layers of the aura. These crystals operate at a higher level of consciousness, thereby bringing the harmonic frequencies of the angelic realm into the energy field. The net result brings "the subtle bodies into harmony and activate[s] intuitive rebalancing of the soul body."[44] Terminated crystals of amphibole-included quartz can also be used to sort the information or patterning contained in each of the subtle bodies. This restores balance to the aura by placing the karmic patterns back into the causal body, where they can be naturally resolved.

Russian Lemurian Quartz

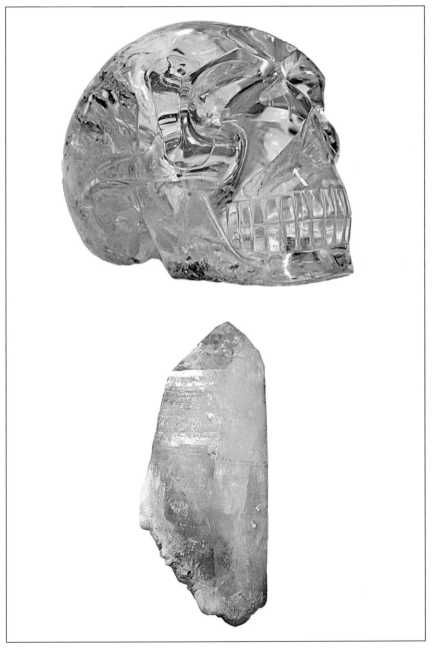

A masterfully carved skull in Russian Lemurian quartz (above);
sacred scribe from the original mine in the Ural Mountains (below)

Available shortly after the initial deposits of Lemurian seed crystals were mined in Brazil, their Russian counterparts have always been in short supply. Russian Lemurian quartz was mined for only a short while, and it typically exhibits a smoky-to-citrine coloration. Many of the crystals were not harvested intact; broken edges and incomplete terminations are the norm for the Russian Lemurian crystals. Although it does not display the same overall morphology of the Lemurian seeds, most Russian Lemurian quartz does tend to exhibit the horizontal striations for which its crystal brethren from Brazil are best known.

These Lemurian crystals hail from the Ural Mountains of Russia; they feel wise, ancient, and holy. Their very presence seems to align and clear the space they are placed in, such that it becomes better attuned to the planet. The Russian Lemurians were named "sacred scribes" by JaneAnn Dow, as they are believed to act as records of all that was and all that will be. The horizontal striations on these crystals occasionally form alongside other interesting etchings and geometric markings. They feel as though they are encoded with a language older than humankind.

These crystals are not karmic healers in their own right. Instead, they lead the way for the consciousness to tap into the prototypic patterning of fulfilling your highest potential. These crystals are aligned with the energies of the Akashic records, and they are powerful teachers for human consciousness. The sacred scribes help you to read the information contained in the records, and they are especially helpful in connecting to your soul contract. Sleeping with one of these crystals can help you sort through outdated contracts in your dream state.

Although these crystals are very rare, a newer variety of Lemurian quartz has recently been made available to crystal healers. These brilliantly clear chunks of quartz are named Lemurian ice quartz for their resemblance to frozen water. They are only available as irregular pieces in lieu of terminated crystals. Many are optically clear, and they are frequently graced with luminous rainbows. The energy of the Lemurian ice quartz is decidedly more mental than their sacred scribe cousins.

They can be placed at the causal chakra or at the base of the skull in order to help the higher mind integrate its causal awareness into the lower mind.

Lemurian ice quartz brings a technical, methodical, almost impersonal energy to us as we ready ourselves for evolution. Like other Lemurian crystals, they, too, are seeded with ancient wisdom from the root race of Lemuria. However, this information is less emotionally centered than most of the analogous crystals found elsewhere. They activate the encoding in our causal body that has lain dormant through most of our lifetimes in order to awaken a greater understanding of the how and why of what is happening in the universe. Holding one in each hand during meditation fosters appreciation for and recognition of the law of cause and effect in action.

Spirit Quartz

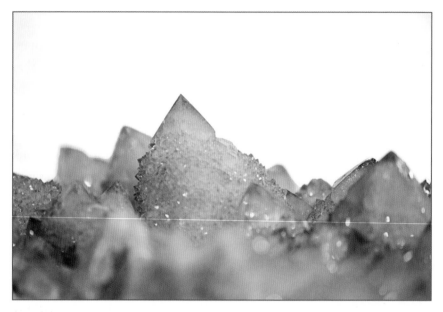

Spirit quartz

Spirit quartz is the trade name for a striking crystal formation that was discovered in South Africa, first appearing around 2001. The crystals, found inside an iron-bearing matrix, resemble a cactus; they consist of a central crystal point with hundreds of tiny crystals growing outward along the six faces of the body of the crystal. These smaller terminations are perpendicular to the growth of the central point, directing their energy to radiate outward in all directions. Due to the presence of iron, these quartz crystals may exhibit any combination of purple, yellow, gold, brown, reddish, clear, and mauve colors. Those examples with purple portions also embody the properties described above in the amethyst entry.

Spirit quartz has a radiative, projective quality. It feels as though it broadcasts its vibrations in all directions, linking together everything within its grasp. It has an uplifting, serene quality that permeates the environment. This special quartz formation also helps to unify separate ideas, energies, and entities toward a common goal or orientation, just as the tiny crystal points align themselves along the faces of the central quartz.

Spirit quartz may help you explore the past-life links you share with those around you. It can help to facilitate spiritual journeys to the Akashic records and maintain a safe environment during past-life regressions. The morphology of this unique quartz reminds us that the soul takes on many incarnations in many eras, including simultaneous ones. It also depicts the way individual soul groups are linked together in a unifying family or monad, as well as the way that monads are also linked higher up in our spiritual makeup. In light of this, spirit quartz facilitates connecting to members of your spiritual family, especially those who may share your karmic burdens so that you can work to release them together.

Spirit quartz is perhaps best suited to releasing and transmuting our family karma, as well as the karma of larger groups such as nations, races, and the planet. Amethystine spirit quartz has been found to be the most effective at this because it burns brightly with the violet flame and directs this spiritual flame to each person represented within a group. Spirit quartz can help to mitigate the effects of past-life karma in the present life by initiating a clear understanding of the how and why of the karmic patterning underlying a present situation.

Adding spirit quartz to any crystal grid meant to release and transmute karma will expedite and intensify the results. It is an able healing stone and helps to cleanse and purify the space in which it is kept. For this reason, this type of quartz is the stone of choice for working on large-scale causal healing.

Time Link Crystals

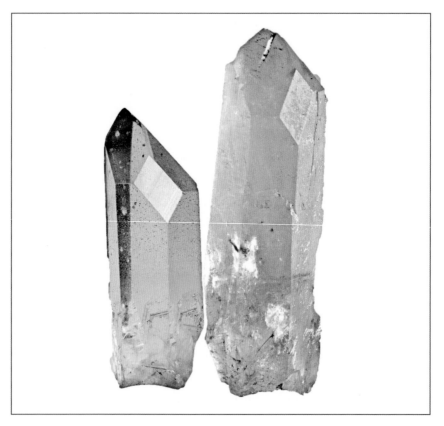

Time links to the past (left) and future (right)

Time link crystals are quartz crystals that display an additional, parallelogram-shaped window near the termination. This extra facet should be centrally located, often just beside the focal point or central face on the crystal's point. Time links are one of the twelve master crystals, a group of special quartz configurations meant to guide the evolution of consciousness.[45] The time link window may slope upward to the right, making it a future time link, or upward to the left, wherein it is a past time link.

Much like the effect of calcite's rhombohedral crystal lattice, described on page 92 in the entry for calcitized shells, the extra face on the time link crystal is a tool for linking parallel realities.[46] One of the lines in the parallelogram is your current reality, and the other long line indicates concurrent lifetimes. The lines at the top and bottom of the face join together events or timelines that ordinarily do not overlap. The crystal therefore serves to dissolve the awareness of time as being purely linear, and can facilitate an expanded awareness through which time is no longer viewed as a limitation or setback.

Placing the time link facet against the third eye or heart, or even gazing into it, will initiate past-life recall or shamanic journeying to observe concurrent lifetimes. Time links do more than simply facilitate the journey; they actually work toward helping you recognize your former self at the soul level, as well as integrating the experience and lessons of a particular lifetime.[47] The extra face, with its elongated appearance, is akin to a "ribbon of light" programmed to enable time travel.[48]

Unlike most other past-life stones, the time link crystals go one step further: they permit you to rewrite and reframe your soul's history. This can clear patterns of karma at their inception, thus erasing the influence of a karmic pattern from all subsequent timelines. These crystals are potent catalysts that propel our evolution toward achieving perfection by endowing us with an opportunity to rewrite our soul's history and future. Meditating and journeying with time links can offer a chance to communicate directly with a past or future incarnation in order to gain clarity and insight into your current scenario. This can help you merge otherwise divergent and disparate aspects of the self into one whole, integrated self.

Trigonic Crystal

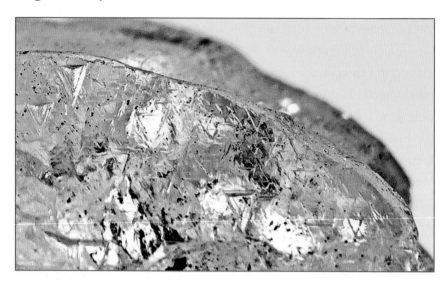

Trigonic quartz displaying downward,
triangular glyphs

When quartz, or any other mineral, displays triangular etchings, apparently incised into the surface of a crystal face, these are called trigons. Trigonic etchings were apparently quite rare several decades ago, and they are becoming more readily available today. Trigonic crystals differ from record keepers in that the triangular markings are always sunken into the face, as though carved, and they always have the point facing downward. Although they share similar effects with record keeper crystals, they work on a transpersonal level rather than an individual level.

The trigonic crystal is an initiation stone; it facilitates transcendental experiences and opens cosmic doorways to higher consciousness. The geometric markings on these crystals resemble the type of patterning in the aura that expresses the blueprint of the soul. Trigonic crystals are the "midwives of the soul," and they can facilitate any journey made by the soul, such as birth, death, and spiritual journeying.[49] The etchings on these crystals "represent the connecting link between the physical consciousness and our superconsciousness, or oversoul expression."[50] This crystal actually reaches out past your personal blueprint into the level of organization of the oversoul or monad. It facilitates out-of-body travel and transpersonal, spiritual experiences. The trigonic crystal is not necessarily healing at the lower levels; instead, it assists in the integration and understanding of soul blueprint information. It can be used to set or fix a fledgling pattern or cycle that is helpful to your growth or healing process by connecting that pattern directly to your spiritual encoding.

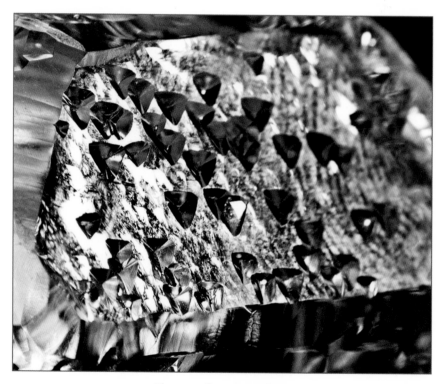

Close-up of trigonic etchings

Trigonic quartz is aimed at soul-level healing. For this reason it belongs to the family of healers in which the diamond is grouped. In fact, natural diamond crystals often exhibit the same trigonic etchings. Trigonics can heal and rectify the spiritual blueprint as well as catalyze the expression of it here in the third dimension. Trigonic crystals are some of the most powerful crystals available in that they can affect the fabric of the soul and its spiritual patterning. Trigonic crystals are guides and teachers that help one explore the many aspects of creation and more fully express one's inherent connection to Source.

RHODOCHROSITE

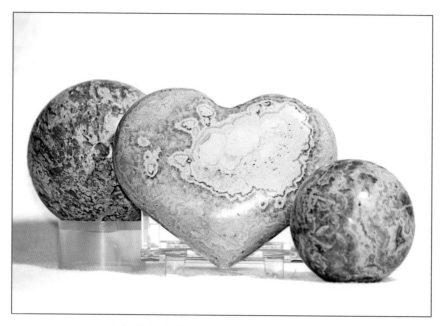

Polished rhodochrosite from Argentina and Peru

Sometimes called "Inca rose," rhodochrosite is a carbonate of manganese, varying in color from white and pink to shades of peach, orange, and red. It is a softer stone, and it is found in Colorado, Romania, Germany, Argentina, and South Africa. It forms crystals similar in appearance to calcite, such as scalenohedrons and rhombohedrons, and the two minerals form within a single series.

Rhodochrosite brings freedom of spirit to its owner. Fine, gemmy pieces of rhodochrosite display an orangey, red-to-pink color that vitalizes the energy field enough to break free from restricting patterns. It brings joy, freedom, and mirth when used in crystal healing, and it helps to nourish and encourage the inner child. It is used to release childhood trauma such as any causal pattern beginning in childhood. This is inclusive of karma initiated during early years in concurrent lifetimes, too. It eases the emotional side of the karmic pattern, thereby making it easier to let go and move on.

To the Inca of South America, rhodochrosite was believed to be "the solidified blood of their ancestral kings and queens."[51] It can help heal the karma of our ancestors, which is sometimes inherited upon incarnation. It responds to the weight and fear often ingrained into these causal patterns by means of love and compassion. The pinkish, peachy colors in rhodochrosite bridge the heart and solar plexus chakras, which enables this crystal to activate the sense of will and personal power through love and kindness.

Rhodochrosite creates a whirling energy that clears and reorganizes the causal and emotional bodies. It can help to separate the energies that may have been misplaced in the aura's different strata. By returning causal energy back to the causal body and emotional energy into the emotional body, one can more readily observe, analyze, and act on the information about karmic patterns. This in turn can assist in decision-making and follow-through in a variety of avenues in life.

Wearing rhodochrosite improves and stabilizes changes in your life. It fosters a sense of self-confidence, which helps mobilize and motivate you to break free from limiting energies, including causal patterns. It is an ideal stone for overcoming self-doubt originating through childhood programming, and it can help to wipe these ideas and their causal counterparts away, leaving a template of confidence in their stead. Rhodochrosite brings a sense of loving-kindness to the activity of change, which allows one to gently but assertively make the necessary changes in overcoming negative mental and emotional cycles and to break bad habits, some of which may result from residual karmic energy.

SELENITE

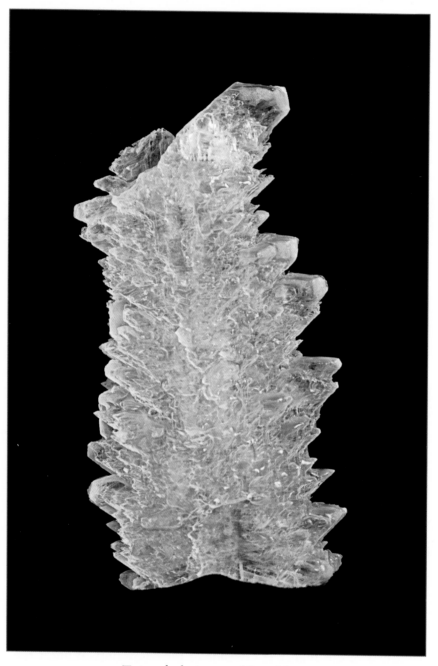

Twinned selenite crystal from Mexico

Selenite is the name given to crystalline, lustrous forms of the mineral gypsum. Gypsum is a very soft, porous compound containing a sulfate of calcium and water. It crystallizes in many shapes and colors, and selenite as a whole is a stone of activating our connection to our higher selves and to Source. It is a tool for raising consciousness and learning to better embody the light of your divine self. Given that selenite forms as water evaporates, it often contains a strong link to the water elements and the emotional body.

Selenite is the main activator for the soul star chakra, a beacon of high-consciousness light.[52] Selenite bursts open the doors to the higher self, making it is an invaluable tool for crystal toolboxes. Selenite's brilliance and luminosity is countered by its physical softness. It is both forceful and gentle, and this variable nature allows it to unlock areas of the subconscious that may not respond to other tools or techniques. Selenite also has a very cleansing energy overall. Sweeping it through the aura can help to release karmic debris, and it can be placed on an energy center in order to purge it of stagnant programming. Selenite works through its relationship with light, both physically measurable light frequencies and the spiritual light. It is naturally fiber-optic and conducts light to any place in need of it.

Selenite is a quickly forming mineral, sometimes cropping up in flooded mines just short periods of time after miners leave. It can take unusual shapes, such as curved and spiraling crystals, and it may exhibit unique phantoms and color zoning. Selenites from around the world are beautiful and versatile tools. Although selenite does not resonate directly with the causal body, it does direct higher planes of light and consciousness into the causal chakra. In this manner it initiates contact with higher beings, the angelic realm, and our own souls. Selenite awakens us to the higher, greater reality of who we are. As spiritual beings we are only temporarily coming into physical incarnation in order to learn karmic lessons. Selenite thus permits us to experience the wholeness of our higher self outside of the constraints of linear time and causal patterns.

Black Phantom Selenite

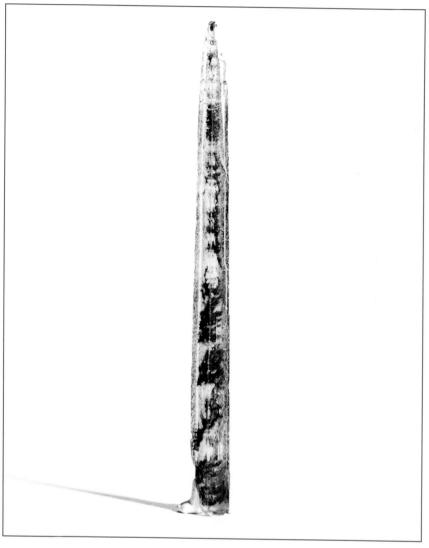

Australian black phantom selenite

Black phantom selenite occurs in several crystal forms and is mined in a few locations around the world. Thicker, striated crystals with patchy, dark inclusions are more typical of finds in Mexico. Tapered, blade-like crystals of selenite from Australia occasionally form with layered phantoms of black inclusions, too. In either case, the white light of selenite's energy is balanced with the dark phantoms contained within. All phantom crystals are excellent tools for exploring past lives and their lessons. Selenite phantom crystals exhibit similar properties, and they contain the additional effects of the selenite out of which they are formed.

Black phantom selenites are typically powerful tools for bringing light into the shadows. The Mexican variety resembles a pillar of light, with shadows suspended within it. The activity of these crystals works in a similar fashion. Connecting to these powerful allies results in an encapsulating effect; they inundate our shadow aspects with so much light that they are broken down and carried away. These crystalline allies can be consciously directed to transmute the karma that we have carried from this and previous lifetimes in order to leave us feeling lighter, freer, and more vibrant.

When you have access to thinner, terminated examples of black phantom selenite, they make excellent tools for hands-on healing. The sharp points and well-defined edges result in a tool that is capable of cutting away karmic debris and slicing through energetic cords. Using crystals in this fashion requires sensitivity and caution, for it is necessary to patch up and nourish the area receiving these treatments. Whenever cords or other energies are removed from the aura, the surrounding area is vulnerable to outside influences, as is the case with physical surgery. The auric opening can be closed by using your selenite crystal to project light and healing into the space until it is fully saturated. Afterward, apply one of the gemstones that nourishes the aura, such as golden beryl, as well as an overall healing and nurturing stone, like rose quartz. These stones help anchor the positive changes that have been enacted, thus making them strategic partners for such applications.

Occasionally, through a process called parallel growth, multiple, smaller terminations will cascade down from the main point of a crystal. When this happens with black phantom selenite, such as the

Australian type, the crystal may vaguely resemble a key. These crystal keys can be applied to the subtle anatomy in order to unlock karmic debris being held within the physical and spiritual bodies. Approach the aura gently and bring the crystal into the field of the heart center. By gently turning the crystal (you'll need to check to see which direction works), you can release trapped causal energies, helping them return to their source for remediation.

When the crystal is gently pulled away, the energies of karma will be drawn away with it. Imagine a safe place for this karmic programming to go, such as a vessel containing the violet flame. It is imperative to erase or transmute this energy before proceeding in order to prevent anyone from accepting another person's karma.

Hourglass Selenite

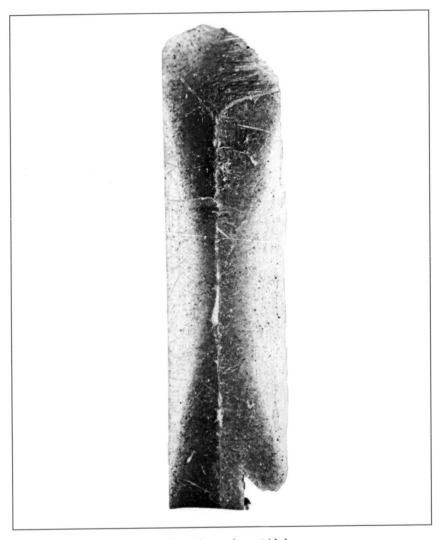

Hourglass selenite from Oklahoma

These unusual selenite crystals are found in Oklahoma, in the Great Salt Plains lake bed. They display an hourglass-shaped inclusion composed of embedded grains of sand. These blade-like minerals are discovered just below the surface of the salt plains, and the fineness of the sand correlates with the clarity of the mineral specimens.

Hourglass selenite contains a striking inclusion, and just like the sand in actual hourglasses it gives these crystals an interesting relationship to time. The grains of sand are frozen in place within the selenite, seemingly implying a state of timelessness. Meditating with these gypsum crystals cultivates better awareness of the present moment. Since selenite is so intimately associated with optics, these petite crystals remind us that the fabric of time, as well as space, is held together by the realms of light, just like the particles of sand maintained within hourglass selenite.

Moreover, the incredible symmetry of the hourglass inclusions in these selenite crystals embodies the spiritual axiom "As above, so below." They point us toward recognizing that our intrinsic perfection is genuinely unaffected by causal energy. In this way we can shed our karma and return to the grace of divinity with which we are created. Hourglass selenite initiates communion with the higher self in such a way as to help manifest change at that level; this, in turn, results in lasting, and often immediate, change here in the physical world. Combine these crystals with other karmic healing stones to illuminate and disintegrate the causal baggage that is being carried.

SERPENTINE

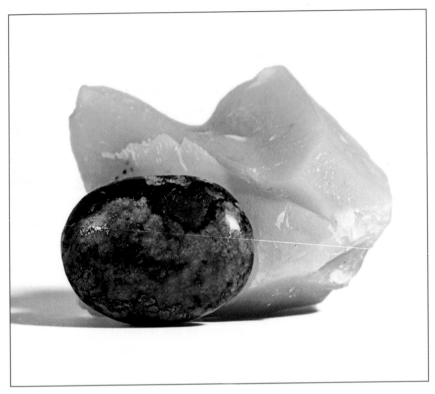

Tumbled serpentine

Serpentine is a family of rock-forming minerals, each of which has a fibrous structure and contains iron and magnesium. Named for its generally greenish color, serpentine can form as compact masses, asbestiform fibers, and in a mixture with other minerals. Serpentine minerals usually range in color from green to brown, although they may also be gray or black. They may also be patterned, such as with spots or stripes. Serpentine is sometimes sold as "new jade" and often resembles jade, although it is much softer and easier to carve.

Serpentine is very peaceful, not unlike jade. It can facilitate movement, such as by promoting flexibility in the body or by helping stagnant energy return to a state of flux. It is therefore also used in activation and awakening of the kundalini, the "slumbering serpent" of energy that climbs through the central column of our energy body when activated. Serpentine is a helpful adjunct to integrating stones that have difficult lessons; it helps by bridging where we are currently vibrating and where the stone would have us be after its energy has been integrated.

Connecting to serpentine in meditation is like holding a history book of planet Earth in your hands. It is intimately linked to the consciousness of the kingdoms of nature: mineral, plant, animal, and devic.* It is soothing and quiets the mind and emotions in order to allow the spirit to flow more easily. In doing so, it helps to "unlock the stored cumulative knowledge of the natural world."[53] In its own way, serpentine can thus facilitate past-life recall, especially if lifetimes have been experienced as other forms of life. This can enrich the time we spend here in our human forms by offering a glimpse into the miracle of being human.

Serpentine is geared toward growth and rejuvenation. It promotes cellular regeneration and can ease joint pain and improve spinal alignment. It can also help release conditions related to karma by letting one's spirit explore the previous lifetimes in which this karma has been created.

Magnetite often occurs as inclusions in serpentine, especially chrysotile, an iron oxide that is highly magnetic. Magnetite balances opposite polarities, confers grounding, and is extremely helpful for protection and guidance. It is an excellent stone for accessing the Akashic records. Combined with serpentine, "it acts as a recorder of Earth changes and Earth shifts as told through the geological and energetic patterns of this metamorphic stone."[54] This helps to guide us on our path by enabling humankind to learn from previous changes and transitions. Among these occurrences are a number of cataclysmic events that have negatively imprinted the causal bodies of many people. Combine this rock with amethyst or opal to purify the karmic baggage centered around these causal patterns.

Devic is derived from the Sanskrit *deva,* meaning "heavenly" or "divine." Devas are the conscious, personified forces of nature, and they dwell in the devic plane or realm, a level of reality just outside our own. They are responsible for maintaining the balance of the natural world and all it contains.

Atlantisite

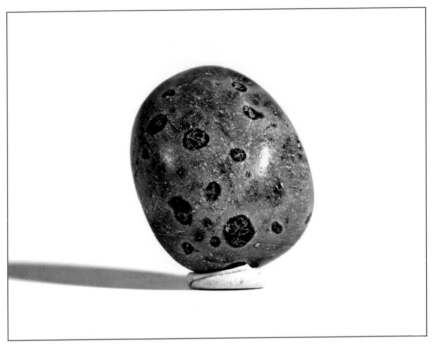

Atlantisite displays purple inclusions of stichtite in green serpentine.

When bright-green serpentine occurs with inclusions of stichtite that are visible as purple patches, it is often referred to as Atlantisite. It combines the energies of serpentine with those of stichtite. It is considered to have an effect that curbs the impact of the negative karma incurred during the Atlantean civilization, from which it derives its name. During the peak of Atlantean civilization, it is believed that the populace of Atlantis began to misuse its power and technology. Many believe that it was a misuse of crystal technology that incited the fall of Atlantis. After the fall, human consciousness was set back; spiritual gifts went into hiding as the secrets of Atlantis sank beneath the waves. Atlantisite accomplishes its healing mission by combining "the vibrations of love, forgiveness and spiritual illumination, linking the heart and crown chakras."[55] By linking emotional and mental energies together in a manner conducive to growth, Atlantisite can undo the wounds of hubris incurred during the Atlantean era.

Working with Atlantisite is calming, and it combines the past-life recall of serpentine with the violet energy of stichtite. This allows it to carry the violet flame directly into past-life experiences for karmic resolution. Atlantisite partners well with record keepers in order to activate a clearer vision of life in Atlantis for teaching purposes. It can also be used in conjunction with Lemurian seed crystals in order to restore the balance between the archetypal energy of the lost root races of Atlantis and Lemuria.

Chrysotile

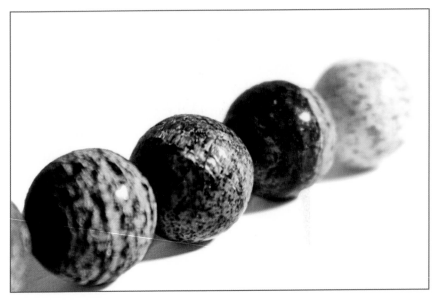

*Chrysotile's fibrous structure
often displays chatoyancy.*

Chrysotile is a specific member of the serpentine group, and it is frequently available as striped masses of green stone. It is the "keeper of the soul's contracts," and it is helpful when placed at the causal chakra.[56] Chrysotile invites your consciousness to step into a different timeline altogether, wherein the effects of previously held karma are lessened or altogether neutralized. This can help in rewriting your soul's contract and sidestepping the patterns set up to play out in your causal body.

Chrysotile can be brushed through the aura at approximately the height of the causal body to loosen karmic debris that is in conflict with your purpose or mission in life. Combined with Welo opal in particular it will disintegrate this causal energy through the incendiary properties of the opal. Chrysotile will locate the outdated patterns and agreements so that the opal can burn them away, leaving you feeling freer and more vibrant.

SHUNGITE

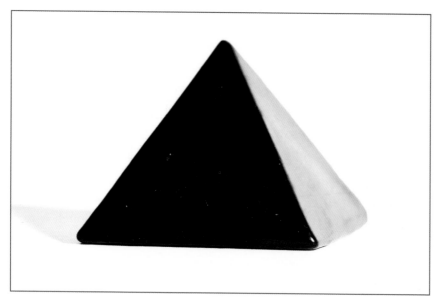

A polished shungite pyramid

Shungite has risen in popularity quite rapidly since its introduction to the world of crystal healing only a few years ago. It is a carbon rock from Karelia, Russia, that contains fullerenes: special and complex molecules of carbon-shaped tubes. Although it is a relative newcomer to the rest of the world, in Russia shungite has been a traditional remedy for conditions of the skin, inflammation, pain, and sickness in general. Now it is being recognized as the most efficient and powerful tool for preventing or reducing the negative side effects of harmful electromagnetic field (EMF) exposure.[57]

Shungite, being mostly carbon, is a powerful stone for bodily healing. It is strongly grounding without ever endowing a sense of heaviness or slowness that other grounding stones can offer. It is excellent for sensitive people, as it helps to filter out disharmonious energies from many sources, including other people's emotions. Shungite has the ability to catalyze purification; its energy sweeps through the physical and nonphysical bodies and helps to release trapped energy patterns from the most basic units of our existence.

Although its effects are not specifically geared toward releasing and purifying our karma, it is powerful when paired with other gemstones whose focus is on the causal energies. It makes a diligent partner to stones such as opal, rhodochrosite, wind fossil agate, and other karmic healers because it sweeps away the patterns of karma revealed by these gems. Shungite's composition enables it to refine its focus at the level of our physical embodiment. It can guide the energy of other gemstones deep into our cells and our DNA in order to sweep out the imprint of negative karma from our entire being.

Because shungite is such a protective stone, it can also be applied toward preventing the uptake of new karmic cycles. Although it cannot stave off the negative effects of your own decisions—it isn't a "get out of jail free" card—it can certainly prevent you from accepting more negative karma than you have actually earned. This includes settings in which you are offering healing to others; instead of accepting the karmic patterns you facilitate others in releasing, shungite guards you from taking on what isn't yours. Its grounding effects can also be used to center the mind and offer clearer thinking, which can help you make the right decisions to prevent creating new karma, too.

SODALITE

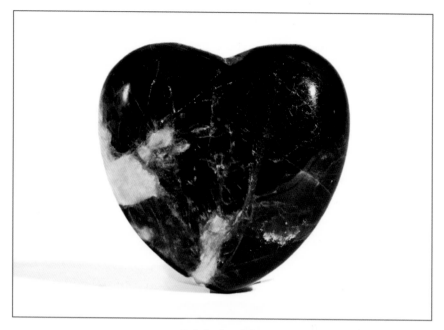

Polished sodalite

Sodalite is a commonly available gemstone, and it is found in several locations in a continuum of grades, from opaque pale stones to rich indigo stones approaching transparency. Sodalite refers to a whole group of rock-forming minerals, including the lazurite from which lapis lazuli is formed. The most abundant member of this family, the eponymously named sodalite, is usually opaque and exhibits patches of white. Sodalite is a member of the cubic crystal system, and its name and color result from its sodium content.

Sodalite has a purifying effect. It helps to clear stagnant energy in the mental body, and it also clears blockages in the throat and third-eye chakras. It can be used to eradicate persistent thoughts underlying behaviors that when left unchecked become negative karmic patterns. Sodalite helps to inhibit negative karma through preventive care.

The finest sodalite is more observably crystalline; among gemstones it is recognized as the official carrier of the indigo ray.[58] This type of sodalite is translucent to transparent and often forms as portions of masses containing the typical white impurities. As the anchor for the indigo ray, sodalite rules over the domain of Saturn in our physical body: the skeleton, teeth, ligaments, cartilage, and joints. The cubic geometry of its molecular organization further emphasizes this energy of form and structure. It helps to ground the spiritual world into the material world. This makes it an excellent stone for those trying to combat materialism, especially by divulging any karmic patterns that may have instigated it. It especially helps by revealing a more spiritual point of view.

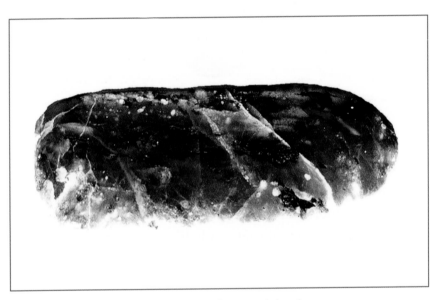

Gem-quality translucent sodalite from
the Princess Sodalite Mine in Bancroft, Ontario

Saturn rules the passage of time and the reaping of what you sow; given this, the carrier of the indigo ray, sodalite, gives access to the nature of your life purpose and the spiritual structure beneath what we experience in life. It may give a step up in peeking into the information stored at the blueprint level, although it does so indirectly. The indigo color of sodalite awakens the inner sight by activating the third eye. It can help clarify psychic vision and enhance the recall of dreams. This other reality, the dreamtime or psychic reality, is the level at which karma is processed on a daily basis. Sodalite entrains you to have a better grasp of the karmic patterns through heightened intuition and more vivid dreams.

Sodalite containing hackmanite, such as material from the Princess Sodalite Mine in Bancroft, Ontario, has an additional karmic effect. Hackmanite is another member of the sodalite group, and it opens the doorway to understanding any scenario from the soul level; it therefore assists in finding the gift in every karmic opportunity.[59] In lieu of viewing challenges as obstacles on the path, this special type of sodalite provides a more optimistic approach, wherein each lesson in life is an opportunity to grow through learning a new teaching. Such stones help us look for the purpose of every event in relationship to the soul.

WIND FOSSIL AGATE

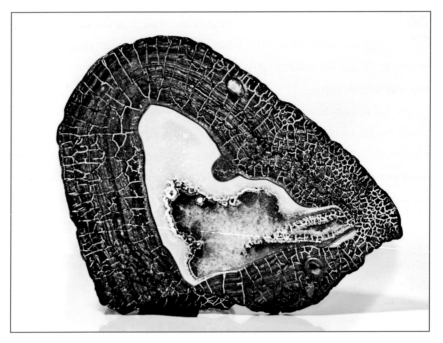

A polished slab of wind fossil agate

Uncommon among agates, wind fossil agate forms as weathered nodules bearing records of their long histories. Judy Hall writes that this stone "symbolizes layers scoured first by water and then by strong winds blowing through desert canyons, leaving the tougher portion prominently displayed."[60] Its appearance combines the usual layered or banded structure of agate with a web of fissures and cracks from being eroded by the elements. The elemental energy that gave rise to wind fossil agate is ever-present when you hold this stone in your own hands. It has an abrasive quality, not unlike the combined sun, wind, and sand that shaped it, and it can break through the layers of confusion surrounding your karma. It helps you to find beauty in the midst of change, for transformation does not always feel graceful. This crystal shares its empathy for our human struggles because it has faced its own.

Much like the action of banded opal, wind fossil agate reveals the karma we are experiencing by highlighting it within the causal body. Because the agate is denser and more crystalline that opalite, it can move with more vigor and determination. It reveals soul contracts, karmic cords, and the emotional baggage that is karmic in origin. This stone is truly a survivor, and it "shows you the karmic strengths that you have to draw on, the survival skills you have developed and the endless possibilities of your soul."[61]

If the energy of wind fossil agate seems too rugged for your healing process, couple it with pink opal to add more grace to the mix. It also pairs nicely with Welo opal, which stimulates a total reframing and release of karma. It can also assist in locating structures of the aura that stem from old karmic patterns; use flint or selenite to cut these away in order to free yourself from persistent cycles once and for all.

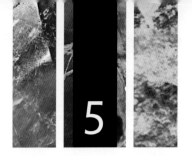

KARMIC TOOL KIT

Putting the Crystals to Use

TODAY'S GLOBAL COMMUNITY of spiritual practitioners, light workers, and healers has access to more minerals than ever before. Hundreds of books describe their properties and applications, although many leave crystal lovers wanting to know more of the "how" once they understand the "why" of crystal healing. Accordingly, the final chapter of this book is dedicated to hands-on applications for anyone interested in healing and transforming karma, including personal, family/ancestral, and planetary.

These techniques are a collection of original innovations and reworkings of more traditional approaches to working with crystals and gemstones. They are meant to be starting points for you in your own journey through causal healing. The methodologies and therapeutic techniques outlined in this chapter are intended to be detailed instructions; however, each application has room for customization and growth. As you deepen your relationship with the mineral kingdom, please feel encouraged to add, alter, and personalize the steps you use to harness crystal power in your life.

The first three exercises in this section are essential preparatory techniques for working with any type of crystalline tool. Familiarize yourself with these steps in order to make the most out of your stones. Following the descriptions for cleansing, programming, and activating crystals, there are a variety of suggestions for how to employ minerals for karmic healing.

Before undertaking any sort of advanced causal healing, establish a good rapport with your gemstones. Treat them with respect, as you would a wise teacher and guide on your spiritual path. Get to know them in meditation; sleep with them tucked beneath your pillow and stow them in your pockets on your daily walk through life. Crystals have more to teach us than can ever be recorded in a book, and the individual stones with which you work are likely to formulate their message and mission for you differently than you might expect. Make your work with them personal and get into the habit of listening to their energies, to their songs.

CRYSTAL BASICS

The mineral kingdom offers some of the most dynamic tools for healing and transformation available to the human race. However, merely collecting and owning crystals is not an effective way to harness their power. It's a little like owning a computer without ever turning it on. Crystals work best when we develop a relationship with them, that is, when we learn to work in tune with them.

Crystals of virtually all types are capable of transmitting, receiving, storing, amplifying, and focusing information, information that is essentially just energy. This means that your most beloved piece of quartz or some other mineral will relay, receive, retain, and intensify the message directed toward or into it. Given that we live in a sea of frequencies swarming around us each day, crystals generally will work with a variety of energies within that spectrum until they are consciously directed to perform otherwise.

When a crystal or gemstone has information or energy imprinted on it that is somehow contradictory to the goal you are trying to achieve, it should be cleansed of the errant vibration. This enables you to start from a clean slate in order to focus on whichever task you have in mind. Remember from the first chapter that crystals are direct incarnations of the divine mind, and when left to their own devices they will always restore a sense of order to their energy. In other words, if we treat crystals as sentient beings, even if they appear to be nonliving matter, their higher intelligence will commence with its ordinary regulatory functions, ultimately resolving any conflicting energy or information contained therein.

This model of crystals as sentient co-creators rather than as inert tools differs from the point of view offered by many previous works on crystals. Describing how this self-regulatory feature works is outside of the scope of this book, but a little trial-and-error experimentation combined with patience will prove it to be true. Remember, the mineral kingdom lives a life measured in geological time, much slower than what we humans experience. Because of this disparity it may appear that some stones need more frequent cleansing, and functionally this will serve as truth, especially in a therapeutic scenario where the same stones will be used for several different clients. In these instances it is necessary to remove the leftover energy, or information, with which the stones may have been imprinted after each client.

There are as many different ways to cleanse crystals as there are people who work with them. Different schools of thought prescribe sunlight, moonlight, salt, water, burying in the earth, placing atop other crystals, sound, chanting, smudge, breath, and prayer, to name just a few. Each method of cleansing your stones will work, especially when you *believe* that it will work. Consciousness is the master of reality, after all.

Many stones are susceptible to being damaged by certain methods of cleansing. As an example, selenite and halite are water-soluble, and amethyst can fade in sunlight. It is imperative that one have a good working knowledge of the hardness, composition, and structure of a stone before engaging in such cleansing procedures. Alternatively, you can choose to practice a safe method of cleansing that will not endanger any crystal, methods that might involve sound, prayer, smudge, or the breath.

In addition to cleansing, programming is an important step in co-creating with the mineral kingdom. To program a stone is to ask it to focus its attention on a specific activity or outcome. A crystal or gemstone that has not been programmed may respond to a given scenario with any number of responses, some of which may not be predictable. With a stone that bears many different therapeutic properties such as quartz, the stone may apply any or all of these benefits to every situation. Amplifying the message or the pain, or transmitting fear are counterproductive but are possible effects when wearing a stone without any conscious attunement or direction.

Programming requires the conscious mind to focus unilaterally on the specific intention you have for co-creating with a given stone. More advanced methods of programming will guide the participant into a higher state of consciousness, wherein the ego mind is bypassed altogether. Either way, the outcome is similar: imprinting a crystal or gemstone with a specific goal. This allows you to direct the outcome of working with gemstones more clearly. Programming works to dial the stone into the frequency you'd like to have broadcasting into your space or your aura, much like tuning the dial on the radio.

Finally, I'd like to touch on the subject of activation. Although some readers may be familiar with charging or empowering crystals, this usually falls into a category that overlaps with one or both of the above topics. Instead, activation is a means to increase the amplitude of the signal being beamed out by your gem. Cleansing wipes away other programs or energies that interfere with your goal, and programming tunes the stone to a particular "channel"; activation raises the volume of that channel in order to increase the likelihood of it being heard.

Activating can also be achieved through a variety of means. I choose to use a method that combines the breath with a focused intention or visualization, and it is very similar to the cleansing and programming methods that will be detailed in this chapter. Each of these methods is based on the work of the late Marcel Vogel, a former IBM scientist turned crystal healer.[1] His methods combine science and spirituality in order to co-create with crystals effectively and efficiently. Vogel has inspired generations of crystal lovers through the legacy of his teachings.

Cleansing Crystals

Cleansing crystals can greatly enhance your ability to manifest and heal with them since it strips away any contradictory or out-of-date programming, as well as any tinge of contamination in the form of other people's vibrations or environmental energy. To practice the method of cleansing inspired by the work of Marcel Vogel, all you will need is a stone of your choice and a space in which you will not be disturbed.

Begin by holding your crystal comfortably in your preferred hand. Terminated crystals can be gently grasped between the thumb and forefinger, if you like. Begin to visualize white light surrounding you, showering down from the heavens and inundating your energy field. With each breath, envision this light penetrating your being more deeply on the inhalation and exhale any vibrations that are not in harmony with the energy of purity.

After several deep, rhythmic breaths, you should feel at ease and clear. Now inhale deeply and connect to your crystal both visually and mentally. Pulse the breath in a series of short, sharp exhalations through the nose, aimed toward the crystal. This breath should be quick and powerful, but it should also be comfortable. It does not serve to make it forced or painful. Visualize the white light being carried on the breath to the stone; picture it sweeping away any discordant or unnecessary information. Repeat for each pair of faces if you like, or merely turn the crystal and repeat on the opposite side.

The idea behind cleansing in this way is that the pulsed breath, when coupled with a consciously directed intention, is very slightly ionized. In doing so, the breath is able to better interact with the crystal lattice from which quartz and other minerals are composed. If your

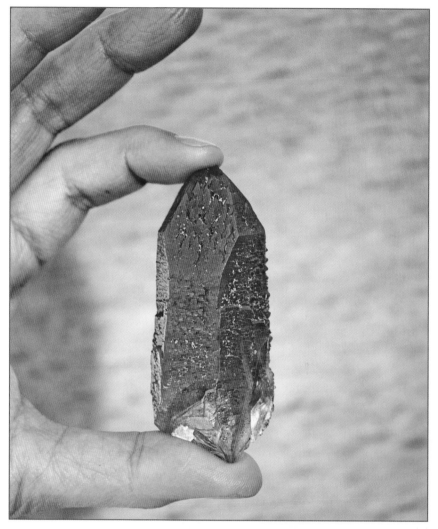

Grasp your crystal between thumb and forefinger.

crystal still feels dirty, heavy, or otherwise impure, refocus yourself and repeat the process.

Programming Crystals

Now that your crystal has been cleansed, it will operate better and be more capable of co-creating with faster, more successful results. However, if you would like to achieve maximum efficiency, programming your crystals is the next step. Choose a recently cleansed crystal or gemstone and prepare for another brief meditation.

As before, hold your stone comfortably in your hand (or hands) of preference. Select an intention or goal that you would like to imprint on your stone. Examples may include broad topics, such as healing, peace, love, wisdom; they may also be more narrowly focused ideas, such as successful past-life regression, releasing karmic debts, erasing soul contracts, and so on. While breathing deeply and in a relaxed fashion, imagine inhaling the intention of your program. Let it fill your entire being, until your body, mind, and spirit are completely resonating with your intention. You may also like to envision an accompanying symbol, word, or color that represents or supports the goal of your program.

Hold the crystal and fill your lungs as you did in the cleansing process. Mentally and visually connect to your stone before releasing the breath in a single pulse through the nose; you may repeat for each pair of faces if you desire. Picture the breath carrying your intention into the lattice of the crystal and imagine that it stays nestled within the structure of the stone. It is a little like downloading a file to your computer so that you can, in turn, use it.

Programming crystals has as much, if not more, to do with the mind than it does the stone. Although asking a crystal to co-create with you for a focused outcome enables it to work toward a specific, reachable target, the greater benefit occurs at the conscious and subconscious levels. In any healing or manifestation endeavor, the greatest enemy is the mind. In cleansing and programming the crystals you are inviting your mind to organize itself toward a precise goal, which reduces the subconscious activity that usually runs counter to spiritual practice. Very often the self is worried about the outcome or it discredits our ability or worthiness for receiving the blessings we are working toward. By engaging with our crystals on such a conscious level and using the kinesthetic approach with the breath, our body, mind, and spirit work together for a common purpose. This aligns and synchronizes our entire being with the programming within the crystal. We are cognizant, conscious co-creators when we program our stones because we finally step out of our own way.

Activating Crystals

Activation of a crystal serves to dial its energy up to its highest potential. Essentially, it is like plugging the crystal into your higher consciousness and all the energy reserves available at that level of existence. Just like the programming exercise, activation really has as much to do with your consciousness aligning and empowering itself as it does the stone. To proceed, pick up your stone, sit or stand in your quiet space, and relax.

To begin, you will need to step outside of your ordinary, waking consciousness. The goal is to bypass the conscious mind by assuming the role of the observer. I usually picture my awareness taking a step backward, behind the awareness of my field of vision. Since the majority of the sensory information that we receive and process about the world around us is taken in through the eyes themselves, by closing them and envisioning moving behind them you can leave the chatter of the conscious mind behind on your spiritual journey.

The next step is to move into a higher state of consciousness now that you are unburdened by the egoic "monkey mind." With the breath, feel yourself rising upward. It may be a sensation of floating or perhaps of riding an elevator or escalator to the next-highest floor in the mansion of your mind. When you arrive at this level of awareness, you will picture being surrounded by a white, brilliant space. It can be visualized as a radiant sphere of light or a luminous room.

Once in this conscious space, project the intention to activate the crystal. Any intention or direction that you hold from this mental place will be magnified, since it is unhindered by the interference of ordinary consciousness. For this reason, keep your focus on simple words or phrases; I generally employ the word *activate*. Let the word and the energy it carries fill the radiant room or space you are in. Just as with the cleansing and programming techniques, breathe in this intention, allowing it to fill your entire being. Connect to the crystal and pulse the activation breath into it.

Activating crystals is recommended for any application with a definite, active goal in mind. It is an essential step in my hands-on healing practice anytime that a crystal tool will be used for cutting through cords or mental patterns, as well as when using a crystal point for any sort of projective task such as long-distance healing, building a protective cocoon, or placing gemstones on target locations. An activated crystal wand is the ideal choice for activating crystal grids or moving and eliminating stagnant energy patterns in a room or human energy field.

One note of caution regarding an activated crystal wand is necessary: proper energy etiquette would recommend that the working tip of a crystal remain covered by the index finger while the crystal is not in use; this prevents it from interfering with someone's personal space or aura. While I do not believe that a properly cleansed, programmed, and activated tool would be likely to cause harm to anyone, it is always best to respect someone's personal space and the integrity of his or her energy field. Be mindful of where you point your crystals! Similarly, when not in use, your wands and other crystals can be stored in a safe place such as a pouch or a padded box so as not to disturb the energy of a space. Many of my favorite stones are on display in my home, but I take extra care not to leave the tips pointing toward where people are likely to sit or stand, unless the stones are part of a healing grid.

When a stone is no longer needed, such as after a healing exercise, it should also be deactivated. This is an easy method to render a crystal back to its quiet, preactivated state. To deactivate a stone, hold it firmly in your dominant hand and "shake it out" just once while pulsing the breath a single time. Merely intend to release the state of activation. This is an easy way to disarm an active stone so that it can be placed innocuously in the environment without disturbing the personal space of anyone or anything without permission.

STONES FOR DAILY WEAR

One of the simplest means of harnessing the power of crystals and other gemstones is to wear or carry them throughout your day. By first cleansing and programming your daily stone, you are inviting it to co-create in a specific manner on your journey. Minerals make for attractive jewelry, and even inexpensive tumbled stones can be worn or tucked into a pocket for an effective tool. After a day of hard work, let your crystal clear itself overnight and restart the process the following day with a new round of cleansing and programming.

The possibilities are endless for which stones you can wear and for what purposes. The combinations are up to you, and your unique vibratory signature will lead you toward certain members of the mineral kingdom that may be more in tune with you. Generally speaking, those stones that feel most comfortable tend to represent the lessons we are most familiar with in life. Crystals that cause discomfort may not be your first choice to wear or carry to work, but they offer tremendous healing opportunities. They feel dissonant because we have not yet integrated their message and energy.

With the above in mind, it is important to match your intention to your desired effect. In all honesty, wearing one of those important, lesson-teaching gems will probably not help you at work or while running errands, even if it is helping you evolve spiritually. Wear more comfortable gemstones while you are out experiencing your normal routine; the challenging stones can be saved for home when you feel less vulnerable. Always try to mentally check in with your state of being in order to decide if the chosen gems are still supporting you and offering harmonious guidance. It may be necessary to remove or cleanse a stone as your day progresses.

The safer, more comfortable choices for everyday wear are explored below. Bear in mind that these suggestions are merely starting points for you to experiment; your intuition and experience are more important than any written guidelines. Resolving and transmuting causal energy can be slow work, but these stones can encourage you and those around you in your daily progress.

✦ **Amethyst** is a great stone for everyday wear, as it is gentle, pacifying, and harmonizing. Program it for anchoring the violet flame so that it can transmute your karma continually. The violet flame will eventually spread through your energy field and begin to heal and alchemize any causal patterns from the environment that it touches. Mix and match amethyst with other karmic healers or blueprint-related crystals in order to blaze and transmute any karma that they help to release.

✦ **Dumortierite** gently moves us forward in life by teaching us to savor the stillness. As much of an oxymoron as that appears to be, dumortierite's message is one of patience. Since linear time is really an illusion, dumortierite helps us to accept the limitless now. This can prevent new causal cycles from being conceived.

✦ **Kyanite** is among the best stones for overall alignment; it has an immediate effect on our nonphysical anatomy, as it restores balance to our auric bodies and realigns our chakras. Since it also activates the causal chakra, wearing kyanite fosters insight into the law of cause and effect that governs the accumulation of karma, both positive and negative.

✦ **Leopardskin jasper** is arguably my favorite stone of all the causal healers to wear all day long. The more you wear this earthy gemstone, the more deeply penetrating its effects are. It gradually saturates your entire aura and aligns you in the flow of the universe, thereby making it easier to attract what you need into your life. By the same token, it readjusts the causal body so that it harmonizes better in your timeline, which can reset any outstanding or stagnant karmic cycles in order to prepare them for release.

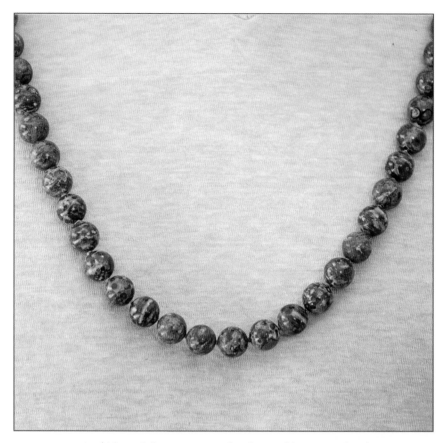

*A necklace of therapeutic-quality leopardskin jasper beads
has a more penetrating effect the longer you wear it.*

✦ **Chrysotile** with **Welo opal** is a dynamic combination. A pendant made of this serpentine with an accent of precious opal will seek out your soul contracts and burn away any that no longer serve you. The process is gentle as long as smaller stones are used, and it can also offer assistance in your relationships. Since the soul's contracts are being continually amended as you wear this combination, it will release any negative karmic ties to other people in your life. The result is more freedom and more room to spread love, rather than pain.

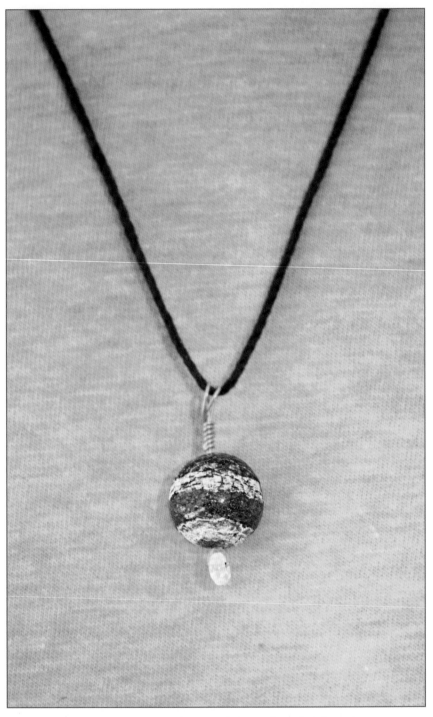

Pendant made from beads of chrysotile and Welo opal

✦ **Shungite** combined with any of the karmic release stones such as **wind fossil agate, banded opal, flint,** or even **aquamarine** will bring refreshing, gentle, and pervasive results. The gem chosen to release your karma will bring unresolved karmic energy to the surface, and the shungite will absorb it like a sponge. The result is deep karmic release with relatively little challenge or emotional pain. Shungite benefits from frequent rinsing in cool water or soaking in the sun; ensure that it is cleansed properly in order to maintain its efficacy.

AWAKENING PAST-LIFE MEMORIES

The past-life chakras are minor energy centers that offer a means of connecting to the accrued lessons of all your concurrent lifetimes. By stimulating these energy centers, which are located at the bony ridge behind the ears, you can bring latent energy to the fore of the mind, which offers greater clarity to past-life exploration and improves your memory overall. Try using these simple techniques prior to a past-life regression in order to increase its efficacy, or use them before bed to recall past-life experiences in the dreamtime.

For this exercise, choose two stones of the same type and approximately the same size to hold at the past-life chakras. Dumortierite, lapis lazuli, Preseli bluestone, and fossils are all good choices. Cleanse your crystals prior to use and program them if you prefer. Lie down or sit in a comfortable position, with one stone in each hand. Take several breaths to relax and set your intention. Move the stones to the past-life chakras and hold the gemstones in place for several minutes. Afterward, relax the arms, holding the crystals in your hands as you proceed into your regression. Alternatively, place them under your pillow when finished if you are using this meditation before bedtime.

Merely stimulating these chakras with the gemstones mentioned above may release or recall past-life information erratically or in brief flashes. Patiently applying the technique over time can fine-tune the

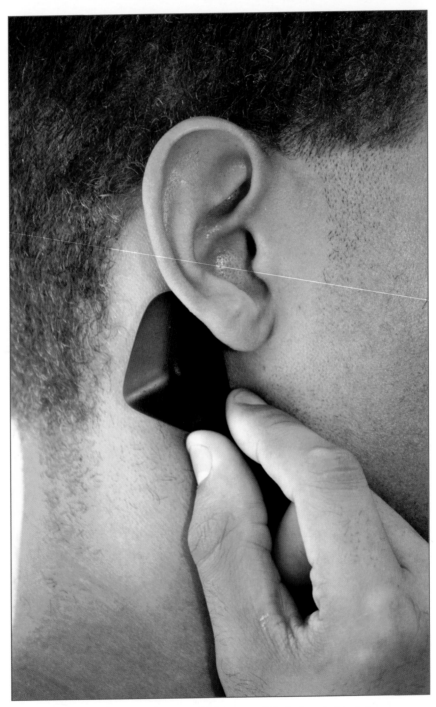

Place your chosen stones on each of the past-life chakras behind the ears.

results. If there is a specific lifetime the memories of which you are trying to access, you can select a guiding stone to place on the third eye or heart in order to direct your meditation toward a recall of that information. Select from the list below or try to match a crystal of your own choice to the lifetime you are hoping to learn from.

CONNECTING TO SPECIFIC LIFETIMES

Certain members of the mineral kingdom share a link to specific times and places in history. When you are aware of karma from a particular lifetime that is in need of healing, using a gemstone as your guide stone can help you to tune in to the specific causal patterns of that life. Generally speaking, the easiest way to match the gem to the target lifetime is based on the provenance of the stone. Select a crystal mined in a specific country or region in order to help alleviate karmic energies associated with a lifetime in that same place.

Additionally, certain types of stones can be used as homing signals for reaching into karma from concurrent lifetimes in particular places and cultures. Many stones that were iconic among some cultures will continue to emit an energy compatible with a bygone culture because the memory is so strong, even if the stone was mined elsewhere. You can combine these gems with any of the other stones used for causal healing in order to fine-tune your efforts to where they are most needed.

The following list is by no means a complete index of stones for specific karmic imprints. Some are not only related to a location or time period but also to other themes or details relevant to a specific incarnation. Careful experimentation, as well as a generous amount of imagination, will allow you to amend this catalog of gemstones to suit your needs. When several ideas are listed for a given mineral, choose the theme or intention that is best matched to the place of origin of your stone. If that information is not available to you, you may simply program the stone to direct its energy toward a location or intention of your choosing.

Many of the stones below are not covered in chapter 4, because they are not necessarily the most multidimensional karmic healing tools. Rather, they work to direct the efforts of the karmic healing stones toward a specific idea or lifetime, and they can be viewed as adjuncts and aids to the healing process. The stones below are listed alphabetically. The most common origins are listed for them, also alphabetically, and for many of the stones additional themes are included. It is not necessary for the past-life scenario and the geographic location to match up in the stone you have selected; simply choose the best options you have available. Be creative when selecting your own stones to connect with specific lifetimes, as there are many more stones that you can add to your karmic tool kit.

Stone	Common Locations	Past-Life Themes
Amber	Baltic States, Russia	Past life during the witch hunts of Western Europe (when combined with jet)
Amethyst	Worldwide	Lifetime spent in the clergy, lifetime with alcoholism, lifetime in seclusion or solitude, spiritual or mystical role
Apophyllite	Brazil, Canada, Germany, India, United Kingdom, United States	Pyramid-building cultures, architecture, construction
Aquamarine	Brazil, Colombia, Kenya, Madagascar, Malawi, Namibia, Sri Lanka, United States, Vietnam	Angelic lifetime
Aragonite	American Southwest, China, Mexico, Morocco, Spain, United Kingdom	Extraterrestrial lifetime (starburst or "Sputnik" clusters only)
Atlantisite	Australia, Canada, South Africa	Lifetime in Atlantis
Basalt	Brazil, Egypt, Hawaii, Iceland, Italy, Russia, United Kingdom	Lifetime as mason or stone carver

Stone	Common Locations	Past-Life Themes
Bloodstone	Africa, Australia, Brazil, China, Czech Republic, India, Russia	Past life as martyr, warrior, or victim; disease connected to past-life injury
Calcite	China, Mexico, United States	Past-life emotional trauma, blocked creativity, or childhood trauma; excellent all-purpose stone for connecting to past life according to location
Carnelian	Worldwide, including Brazil, Egypt, Morocco, United States	Egyptian past life, infidelity, injury or violence
Catlinite (pipestone)	Canada, Minnesota (United States)	Native American culture
Chrysanthemum stone	China	Asian lifetime, gardening
Coral	Worldwide, especially China and Japan	Seafaring lifetime, drowning, connecting to cultures that venerated this stone, such as Tibetan, Nepalese, and Native American incarnations
Cuprite	Afghanistan, Africa, Australia, Austria, Canada, China, France, Germany, Italy, South America, United States	Female lifetime, infertility
Diamond	Africa, India	Lifetime as royalty or ruling class
Eilat stone	Israel, Jordan	Lifetime lived in the Holy Land
Emerald	Africa, Brazil, Colombia, Egypt, India	Lifetime as healer or doctor
Flint	Worldwide	Celtic lifetime, the British Isles, past life as hunter, battle, or war-related karma

Stone	Common Locations	Past-Life Themes
Fluorite	Brazil, China, Germany, Mexico, United Kingdom, United States	Mesoamerican incarnation, lifetime as scholar or philosopher
Fossil	Worldwide	Lifetime as plant or animal
Halite	Austria, France, Germany, Italy, northern Africa, Poland, United States	Lifetime in desert, food-related scenarios, accounting or finance
Iolite	Brazil, India, Kenya, Madagascar, Namibia, Sri Lanka, United States	Lifetime in Scandinavia (especially as Viking), seafaring and navigating experiences
Jade	Australia, Canada, Central and South America, China, Japan, Myanmar, New Zealand, United States	Mesoamerican incarnation; lifetime as artist, artisan, or musician; incarnation as monk, priestess, or clergy
Labradorite	Canada, Madagascar, Scandinavia	Native American (especially Inuit) lifetime, incarnation in other planes, shamanic scenarios
Lapis lazuli	Afghanistan, Egypt, Middle East, Russia, South America	Lifetime as painter or scribe, incarnation as royalty, merchant
Larvikite	Canada, Norway	Scandinavian lifetime, incarnation in cold region
Lava	Worldwide, especially Hawaii and other volcanic locales in the western United States	Lifetime in volcanic region, life lost to natural disaster
Lemurian seed crystal	Brazil, occasionally Australia, China, the Himalayas, Mozambique, Zambia	Lifetime in Lemuria
Malachite	Africa, Middle East, Russia	Death during childbirth
Marble	Greece, Italy, Rome	Lifetime connected to the arts
Meteorite	Worldwide, including the Arabian Peninsula, Argentina, Mexico, Namibia, northern Africa, Russia, United States	Extraterrestrial incarnation, Middle Eastern and Islamic incarnation

Stone	Common Locations	Past-Life Themes
Moldavite	Czech Republic	Extraterrestrial incarnation
Mookaite	Australia	Incarnation in Australia, aboriginal incarnation
Moonstone	Armenia, Austria, India, Madagascar, Poland, Sri Lanka	Lifetime in pre-Christian Europe, as adherent of the Old Religion, motherhood or loss of a child, lifetime as astrologer, diviner, prophet, or priestess
Moss agate	Armenia, Australia, Canada, Hungary, India, Romania, Scotland, United States	Incarnation connected to agriculture, herbalism, or the fairy realm
Nuummite	Greenland	Scandinavian lifetime, lifetime as shaman or astrologer
Obsidian	Central America (especially Mexico), other volcanic regions such as the American Southwest	Lifetime as hunter, shaman, artisan
Opal	Australia, Ethiopia, Honduras, Mexico, Peru, United States	Aboriginal lifetime
Ores (all kinds)	Worldwide	Mining and metallurgy
Pearl	Asia, Oceania	Seafaring lifetime, female incarnation, situations where current illness results from past-life difficulty
Preseli bluestone	United Kingdom, Wales	Lifetime in Celtic culture, Druids
Pyrite	Brazil, Chile, China, Mexico, Peru, United Kingdom, United States	Male lifetime, lifetime characterized by poverty or greed
Quartz	Worldwide	All-purpose stone for connecting to lifetime in any location

Stone	Common Locations	Past-Life Themes
Rhodochrosite	Argentina	Past life in Incan culture, loss of child, childhood trauma
Rose quartz	Brazil, India, Madagascar, South Africa, United States	Loss of loved one, abandonment by partner or family, broken heart
Ruby	India, Myanmar, Sri Lanka	Injury, misuse of wealth or power
Seashells	Worldwide	Seafaring lifetime, lifetime as aquatic organism
Selenite	Common worldwide	Lifetime spent in other plane, beyond physical reality
Shiva lingam	Himalayas, India	Hindu past life, masculine past life, infertility
Sulfur	Greece, Italy, Pacific Ring of Fire, United States	Lifetime connected to fire or ex-communication, being poisoned
Tektites	Australia, China, Indonesia, Ivory Coast, Philippines, Polynesia, Siberia, Thailand, Tibet, United States	Extraterrestrial incarnation
Turquoise	Afghanistan, Africa, American Southwest, China, Egypt, France, Iran, Peru, Russia, Tibet	Native American or Tibetan culture, lifetime as healer or community elder

CUTTING KARMIC CORDS

Whenever you experience an event that impacts you deeply on a karmic level, it is possible for a cord of energy to connect you to the source of the karma. These nonphysical, energetic cords intrude on your spiritual anatomy by burrowing into your aura, chakras, or the physical body, while the other end remains anchored in the person, place, or time associated with the source of the karma. These cords can feed a recurring cycle, thereby making it almost impossible to release the karma without cutting the cord.

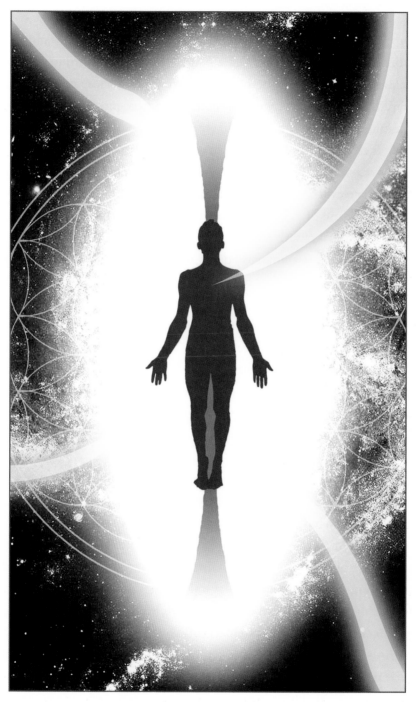

*The aura can host energetic cords linking it
to karmic patterns and memories.*

There are several signs that you may be experiencing a karmic cord. For example, when you change your thoughts, behaviors, or emotions in order to release yourself from a pattern, a cord will continue to feed the pattern energetically despite your having taken those positive steps forward. When events repeat, even after you have integrated the lesson of a causal cycle, then it is also likely you are experiencing an energetic cord. These cords can be trapped in any layer of the aura or any chakra; usually where they are rooted is connected with the type of causal pattern you are experiencing. As an example, a cord stemming from a misuse or underuse of personal power may have one end attached to the solar plexus chakra and the other to the source of your power issues, whether this is a person, place, or point in time. Similarly, emotionally oriented karmic ties may be felt in the heart chakra or in the emotional body in the aura itself.

As trying as karmic cords can be, there is a simple and effective means for removing them. Several crystals are well-suited to cutting through these cords, including laser wands, flint, kyanite, obsidian, and selenite. It is imperative to choose a crystal or stone with a concise termination or sharp cutting edge. Select one that fits comfortably in the hand and ensure that it is cleansed and programmed prior to use.

Begin by holding the intention that you will locate and remove karmic cords. If you wish, call on God, Goddess, Christ, the ascended masters, the angels, or any other positive beings to assist you in the process. Hold the crystal in your dominant hand with the point and base of the crystal between your fingers, if that is comfortable. With a sweeping motion, move the crystal through the aura with the flat side facing you. I usually begin above the head and work downward, moving across the body systematically. In the case of cutting a cord that is behind you, you can ask for assistance in extending your reach spiritually, even if your arms cannot physically touch every part of your energy field. There is no exact sequence to the sweeping; use the motions and directions that are most comfortable for you. When you

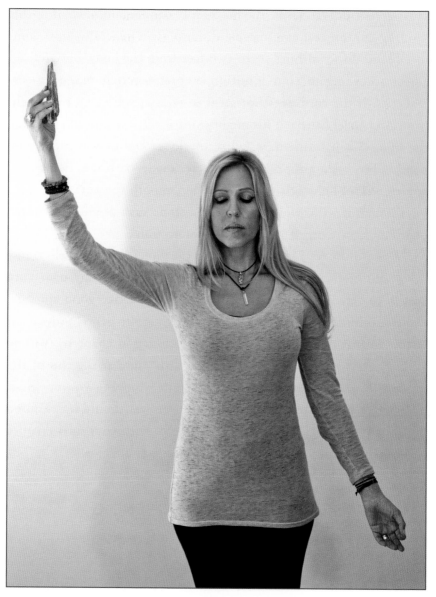

Locating a cord

encounter resistance—which may feel like a change in temperature, a dense spot, friction, or another change in sensation—this is where a cord is located.

Once the cord is located, use a cutting, chopping, slicing, or sawing motion to sever the energetic connection. Perform this severing motion at a comfortable distance. It is generally most comfortable to do so within one to two feet from the body, but you can adjust according to your intuition or preference. It may take several tries. If the cord does not seem to release, you can ask for help from Archangel Michael; his mighty sword will assist you in severing the link. When finished, visualize the loose end of the cord being placed into an appropriate receptacle, made of bright white (or golden white) light or the violet flame. Smooth the aura by sweeping through it with your hand or use a stone such as selenite or rose quartz to help soothe the site of the connection.

When finished, I generally invoke the violet flame to help transmute and eradicate any vestige of the cord within my own aura and in the environment. It is important to practice good spiritual hygiene in order to reduce the amount of karmic debris present on Earth. Any of the masters or angels mentioned in chapter 2 will be willing to assist you in this process. Seal the aura at the end of the process by visualizing a bright white light wrapping you up in an embrace of pure grace and healing. Your crystal should be cleansed immediately by invoking the violet flame or with your own favorite cleansing method.

SORTING CAUSAL PATTERNING

One of the contributing factors to ongoing karmic patterns is causal energy that becomes entangled in the wrong body in a person. Causal energy belongs in a person's causal body, and when it is imprinted or stored in the physical, emotional, mental, or any other body it can lead to illness, unwanted feelings and behaviors, and stubborn karmic cycles that seem to evade resolution. Think of the energy of each of your bodies as being akin to files in a cabinet, each body having its own drawer. If energy is stored in the wrong file, perhaps because we are trying to ignore or repress it, it cannot be healed. An office wouldn't be able to

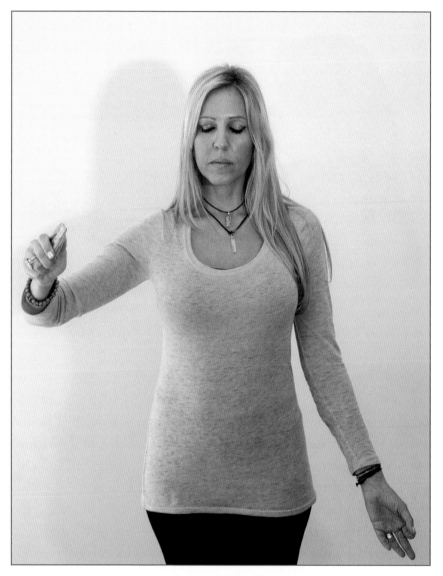

Cutting the cord

accomplish much if its filing system were ignored; your body and aura function similarly.

For this exercise you will need a terminated crystal. I'm partial to the amphibole-included red laser wands and amphibole quartz (described in chapter 4) for sorting the causal patterning in the aura,

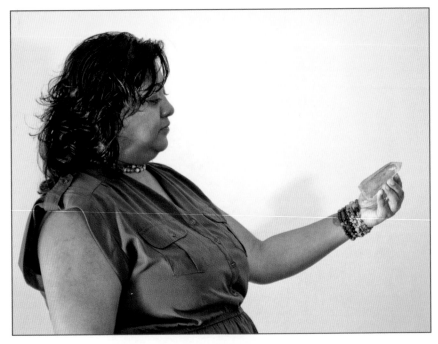

*Begin with the crystal
facing away from the body.*

although many other stones will work, too. A well-terminated elestial crystal, Lemurian seed crystal, or even a polished obelisk of rhodochrosite all serve to accomplish similar results. Cleanse, program, and activate your healing tool before proceeding.

Hold the activated crystal with the base toward the heart and the termination away from the body. Ask that the crystal be guided to any causal patterns that need to be refiled. Sweep the crystal through the aura, beginning close to the physical body; gradually move it farther into the outer reaches of the aura as you progress. I usually sweep from the head downward, but you may follow your intuition to determine the direction and height at which you move the crystal. Permit your hand to be guided in any pattern, direction, or movement as you work. As you go through the many layers of the aura, the base of the crystal is being directed to take in causal patterning from the mental, emotional, etheric, and physical bodies. The karmic

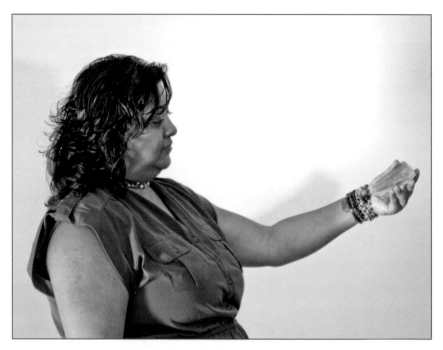

Fill any vacancies you've opened by reversing
the direction of the crystal's point.

energy then travels through the tool and is directed back into the causal body. This helps to restore balance to the function of each of the layers of the aura.

When you feel as though you have completed the task, reverse the crystal, such that the point is directed toward you. Hold the base of the crystal around the level of the causal body, the layer of the aura approximately two-and-a-half to three feet away from the body and repeat the process, moving inward. If the causal body is too far away to reach comfortably, imagine contracting it; see it being pulled closer to your body and into your arms' reach. Hold the intention that any information mistakenly stored in the karmic level of the aura is returned to its rightful place among the other bodies. If you do not sense that this is the case, merely visualize white light filling the vacancies left from the causal energy.

When finished, cleanse your crystal in order to prevent

cross-contamination from the energies it has been moving. Sweep through the aura with an appropriate stone to smooth over the aura and seal up any leaks. Although selenite is my first choice for this, rose quartz, aventurine, pink tourmaline, and hematite may also be used.

GEMSTONE ELIXIRS
FOR KARMIC RESOLUTION

Certain crystals and gems lend themselves to various types of water-based therapies. Any mineral can be used for imprinting water, which can then be consumed or added to bathwater. It's fun to experiment with different gemstones for making crystal elixirs and essences; *be sure to check the composition of your stones first, as some can be toxic.*

It is safest to avoid those rich in heavy metal content, especially the lead stones, including galena, cerussite, pyromorphite, vanadinite, mimetite, crocoite, and wulfenite. Other toxic elements include copper, mercury, nickel, arsenic, antimony, molybdenum, and other metals. It's best to avoid placing minerals with a metallic luster, such as pyrite, lapis lazuli (which also contains pyrite), hematite, galena, or other metallic-looking stones directly in water, as they may release their metal content during the elixir-making process. Soft and soluble crystals such as selenite and halite should not be placed in water, either. These kinds of crystals can still be used with indirect methods of energizing water, even if they cannot be placed directly into the liquid, as described below. When in doubt, always err on the side of caution.

Crystals that are chosen for making crystal elixirs should be physically clean as well as energetically cleansed and programmed in order to provide the optimal setting for effective and safe gemstone-charged water. Containers made from colorless glass work best, although colored glass can be used to harness the effects of color, too. It is best to choose good-quality water, such as spring water, distilled water, or water that is otherwise purified or energized in some way.

Place the vessel with the crystals covered in water in direct sunlight or moonlight and leave it for several hours. In the case of using an indirect method, place the stones in a smaller clear glass cup or container inside the larger clear glass container; water is then added to the outer container without allowing the contents of the smaller cup to come in contact with the water. When making elixirs from combinations that include one or more potentially toxic stones, it is easiest to place all of the stones in the second, smaller container, thus treating them all indirectly.

Once finished, elixirs have a finite lifespan as is. A pinch of natural salt or a splash of brandy or vodka will help to preserve information that has been imprinted in the water. If you plan on drinking the liquid, do so immediately without any preservative. If you prefer to use the elixir as an addition to sprays, baths, or as a topical treatment, the aforementioned preservative can be added in order to ensure a longer shelf life.

Below you will find some specific gems and combinations for treating causal-level conditions. Additionally, you are welcome to experiment in order to discover your own favorite crystal essences.

Aquamarine Essence

Aquamarine essence is the ideal choice for making an elixir that invites energetic liquidity and restores the ability to communicate with the blueprint. Sunlight can cause aquamarine to fade, so choose indirect light or moonlight. It is important to use gems of high quality that have not been irradiated or dyed. The elixir can be enhanced by using a diamond with the aquamarine. If choosing a preservative, a pinch of sea salt is the preferred method.

This gemstone works first at the physical level and gradually detoxifies and resolves blueprint-related conflict on successively subtler levels. It may take several days or weeks to reach the causal level. Consuming aquamarine-imprinted water reminds cells of the perfection in their blueprints and "assists in the transmutation of your DNA into the ideal."[2]

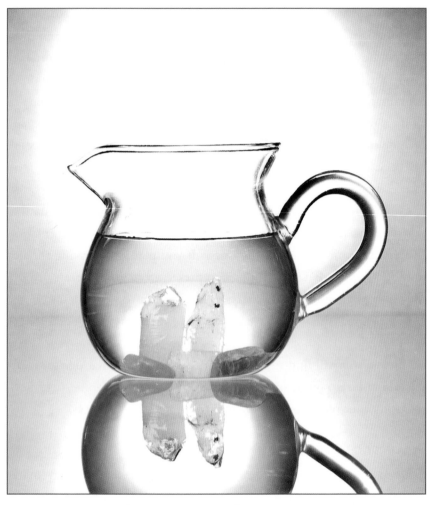

Imprinting water with aquamarine

Aquamarine water may be consumed frequently. Begin with 1 or 2 glasses per day; you may increase the quantity and frequency gradually over time as you integrate the aquamarine vibration and become more energetically liquid.

Karmic Purification Blend

This elixir consists of flint, opal, shungite, amethyst, and red quartz or amphibole quartz. Flint grounds karmic energy, anchors the consciousness, and opens portals through time for the other crystals to work. Opal awakens higher consciousness and helps to resolve karma. Shungite is strongly purifying, and it works with amethyst's violet flame energies to trap and transmute karmic energy. The red quartz (or amphibole-included quartz) serves to burn up negative karma and leave clarity in its wake; if the inclusions form a phantom, it will be even more effective.

This blend is best made by means of the direct method, and either sunlight or moonlight can be used. Take 2 drops under the tongue or gently rub 1 drop on each of the past-life chakras, located on the boney prominences behind the ears, before bedtime.

Soul Journey Blend

This gem elixir strengthens the soul's ability to experience concurrent lifetimes as well as to safely engage in astral travel.

Combine apophyllite, flint, trigonic quartz, and a time link crystal or phantom crystal. Use an indirect method, as apophyllite can be damaged by soaking in water. The quartz crystals can be set up in a grid around the water, if you like; follow your intuition in order to choose the number and pattern of the time links and/or phantom crystals. This elixir is best made with the light of the moon, preferably full, and is preserved with brandy. Take 2–5 drops under the tongue and anoint the third eye with 1 drop before meditation in order to enhance your journey.

Saturn Elixir

To harness the karmic healing powers of the planet Saturn, use the following gemstones: galena, sodalite, and emerald. *It is imperative to use an indirect method for this gemstone elixir, since galena is toxic.*

Galena, as an ore of lead, connects to the alchemically grounding and congealing energy of Saturn. It reflects the nature of any particular cycle in time in order to gain understanding. Sodalite, carrier of the indigo ray, is helpful for fostering the insight and intuition that go hand in hand with a Saturnian comprehension of form and structure; it initiates awareness of the law of cause and effect. Emerald is the truth stone, and in traditional esoteric teachings the emerald color is associated with Saturn; it helps one confront the truth with the heart, and it initiates healing on all levels.

Assemble the stones and begin making the elixir on a Saturday, named for its connection to this planet, and leave the stones in place until the following Saturday. Preserve with brandy or vodka, and use whenever Saturn's help is needed. Take 4 drops before meditation, when you feel ungrounded, want to enhance intuition, or are at the mercy of the inertia of a karmic cycle. It tends to have a slowing effect on circumstances, thereby enabling you to methodically heal or integrate whatever challenge presents itself. Saturn elixir may be used as

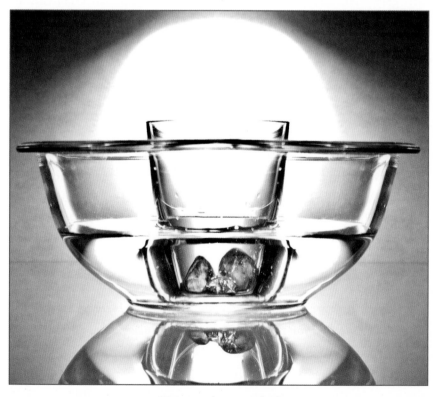

Use an indirect method
to prevent lead contamination.

frequently as needed, but it is best to take it four times a day for long-standing karmic patterns until the scenario is resolved

Releasing Cellular Memory

So much causal information is encoded into our DNA, and it can have a huge impact on our lives. This karma is retained from previous lifetimes and inherited from our family groups. Use amber, amethyst, pietersite, and shungite; they should receive sunlight for at least several hours as they imprint the water. Preserve this blend with a pinch of salt.

Amber awakens cellular memory, and pietersite helps to scrub away causal patterns from the DNA itself. Together, the pairing of amethyst and shungite will scour and transmute the karma that is stored at the cellular and subcellular levels, leaving only life-affirming energy in their wake.

Add 4–7 drops to your drinking water each day for two to three weeks in order to see an improvement. It can also be applied topically to chakras related to any healing opportunities you are undergoing.

Healing the Karma of Illness

It is possible that repeated illness and injury may be remnants of karmic activity. This may be affecting us in the here and now or in other incarnations as well. Combining the following gemstones enables you to heal the patterns of disease on the karmic level in order to restore balance in other affected areas of life: green opal, citrine, shungite, and aquamarine.

Aquamarine helps to detoxify and increase flexibility, including the flexibility of our karmic patterns. Citrine promotes release, and it unwinds the patterns holding the karmic imprint of disease in place; simultaneously it engenders vitality and assists in positive steps forward. Green opal focuses on the karma experienced in association with physicality, including illness. It helps one to see that illness as a learning tool; once the lesson is integrated, disease can be released. Shungite helps to ground the energy of the elixir into the body, and it also supports detoxification and realignment at the cellular and subcellular level, thereby helping the body to reorganize and realign itself toward perfect health.

Take 2–4 drops four times a day under the tongue or place the same number of drops on the site of illness or injury (as long as it won't cause discomfort). You may also add 10–12 drops to the bath, or you can use the elixir as a room spray to help transform the karma being released during the healing process.

Healing Earth's Karma Elixir

The goal of this elixir is to release and transmute karmic debris on a wider scale. It can be sprayed in rooms, around the environment, and around places where many people must pass by. Similarly, a couple of drops can be added to rivers, ponds, lakes, oceans, or fountains in order to disperse its energies around the world.

Combine fossilized wood, selenite, spirit quartz (the amethyst variety), serpentine, precious opal (such as Ethiopian opal), and shungite. Use an indirect method for this elixir, since the selenite and more porous varieties of opal and serpentine will be damaged by submersion. Place the crystals in the container and add the water on the new moon. Leave them in place for an entire moon cycle. Preserve with brandy or vodka and a pinch of sea salt in order to emphasize purification. This mixture can be added to room sprays to clear karmic debris, and it mixes well with essential oils noted for having cleansing properties, such as lavender, cedar, and sage.

RECORD KEEPER MEDITATION

Record keeper crystals are often highly personal meditation tools. While they are usually found as quartz, it is also possible to encounter natural record keepers of corundum (ruby and sapphire), tourmaline, calcite, and diamond, among others. There are multiple methods for accessing the information within any type of crystal, and this method is tailored especially to the record keepers. Alternative methods involve simply meditating with the triangular symbols held against the third eye or heart chakras. Cleanse your record keeper crystal and find a quiet space for meditation. Set an intention, such as retrieving information regarding a specific lifetime or accessing any relevant data that is latent in the crystal.

Take several deep breaths and find an angle that allows you to clearly see the glyphs on the face of your crystal. Let your eyes gaze into one of the triangular markings and begin to relax your focus. As the crystal slides out of focus, allow your eyes to close and let your imagination take over. Continue to picture the triangle on the surface of the stone; visualize it growing larger and larger (see photo on following page). When the etching has grown in height until it is taller than you, imagine it opening like a door.

In your meditation, picture yourself stepping through the crystalline doorway of the record keeper. On the other side you will find the interior landscape of the crystal. You will find yourself in a massive corridor; follow the hallway just within the entrance to the crystal, and it will lead you to a massive hall of records. Use all of your senses to acquaint yourself with the energy and personality of the crystal: What sounds, smells, sights are there within the stone? What is the texture of the walls and floor? What is the taste of the walls of the crystal itself? When you have integrated these sensory elements, your energy field will move into greater harmony with that of the stone.

Inside the hall of records will be receptacles of divine wisdom. These may be books, scrolls, engraved plates and tablets, crystals and gemstones, CDs, or any other type of data storage imaginable. Ask for the crystal to guide you to the relevant information; the consciousness of the stone will direct you to the set of records that you need. If the information appears to be written or recorded in an unknown or

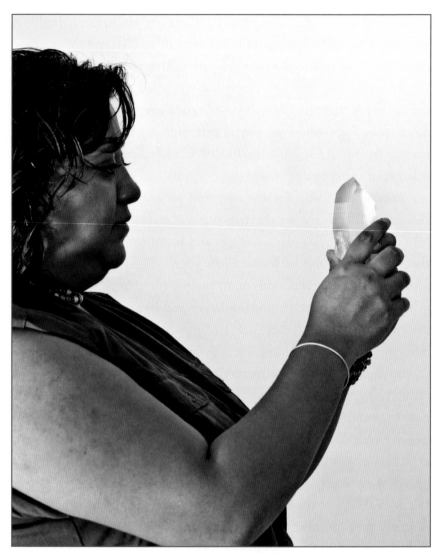

Gaze into the record keeper
and imagine it beginning to grow in size.

illegible script, bring it to your heart center and ask to have the meaning revealed. In this way you can peruse the library contained within the record keeper crystal. Throughout the process, maintain a sense of nonattachment to what you find. Neutrality and objectivity will assist you in receiving the messages of the stone.

When you have obtained the message or information that is desired, restore the records to their rightful places. Thank the consciousness of the stone and return via the same path you originally traveled. Once you reach the triangular doorway, step out and see the crystal shrink back to normal size in your mind's eye. Move the crystal to your heart and picture it permanently copying the information you accessed into your heart center. It will always be available to you thereafter.

PAST-LIFE JOURNEY WITH FLINT

Flint is an ancient stone that has served humankind since the dawn of time. Since it is so intimately connected to human history as a tool, blade, and fire-starting stone, flint can help to guide your consciousness through time to experience an earlier lifetime. Flint is composed of tiny grains of quartz that have replaced lime; it is a recrystallization of once-living material that has evolved into mineral form. Using flint can help you cut through the fogginess surrounding concurrent lifetimes and clarify and ignite the entire journey.

For this meditation you will want to gather two pieces of flint and locate a cozy place to lie down. The first piece of flint will be placed on the earth star chakra to serve as an anchor for the light body as you travel beyond your normal perception of time and space. Flint will also awaken the ancestral memory of your many lifetimes on the planet when placed here. A second piece of flint is placed at the third eye in order to stimulate vision of the concurrent lifetime you will visit. (Placement is illustrated on the following page.)

The first step is to totally relax; with each breath allow your body to free itself of more and more tension. Let yourself feel as if you are sinking or melting into the floor. When you are completely at ease, bring your awareness to your third eye. Visualize your consciousness floating up and away from your physical body. As it rises, let any limiting or disruptive thoughts, emotions, and impulses drift away.

As your consciousness ascends into the ethers, you discover a door

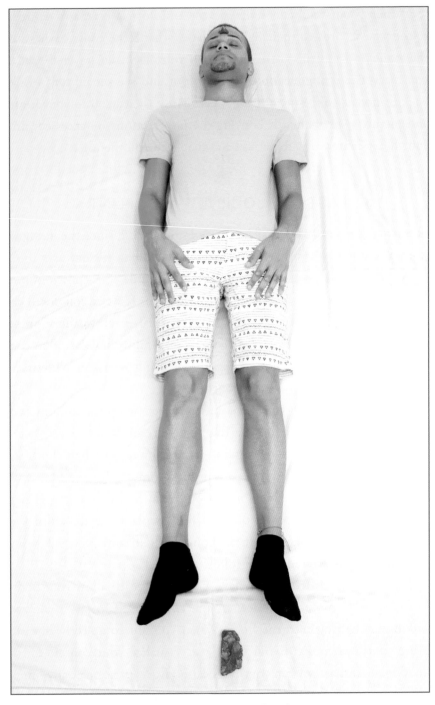

Place the flint as seen in this photo.

awaiting you in the heavens. Open the door and step into the realm beyond it. On the other side of the doorway you find a corridor that stretches to your right and then to your left. The hallway is so long that you cannot see the end in either direction. Lining this hallway are many doors. The doors each represent a specific lifetime, and you will now ask to be shown the lifetime with the most relevant message to integrate.

Follow the hallway toward whichever direction you are led. Soon you come to a door that stands out to you. It may be illuminated differently than the others, or it may be a different color or style. This is the lifetime you are meant to explore. Open the door and walk through to the incarnation on the other side.

At this point, take inventory of the scenario that you see. Some meditators will experience past lives in the first person, whereas others watch them as if on a movie screen. However you experience your other lifetime, try to take in as many details as possible. Consider the following:

- ✦ What gender are you in this life?
- ✦ What age are you?
- ✦ What race or ethnicity are you?
- ✦ In what time period is this incarnation occurring?
- ✦ What are you wearing?
- ✦ Do you recognize any of the people around you on a soul level?
- ✦ What is the biggest opportunity you have to heal by revisiting this lifetime?

However the answers come to you, make a mental note of them without judgment or expectation. Whenever you have seen what you are meant to see, step back through the doorway into the corridor of time. Allow your awareness to be drawn back through the entrance to the hallway and return the way you came. Once your consciousness has returned to your physical body, thank your soul for gifting you with this new past-life insight. If you sense any unhealthy connection between lives such as a karmic cord, you may use the flint to cut this link accordingly.

Other crystals and gemstones can be incorporated into this technique. Preseli bluestone works equally as well as flint, and a time link crystal can be placed on the third eye in lieu of other gems. After visiting concurrent lifetimes to view and learn, you can proceed to apply crystals such as the time link in order to rewrite or reframe the past-life experiences that are still affecting or limiting your current incarnation. For an expanded layout incorporating a more advanced crystal place-ment for past-life exploration, please see the following exercise.

PAST-LIFE REGRESSION CRYSTAL LAYOUT

After becoming familiar with the imagery being used in the previous meditation, an advanced layout can be combined with the journey in order to facilitate releasing and transforming the karmic residue of past lives. As in the previous meditation you'll need space to lie down, as well as the following crystals: flint, petrified wood or another fossil, apophyllite, selenite, and two time link crystals. Additionally, you can fine-tune the journey with one of the stones listed in the "Connecting to Specific Lifetimes" section found on page 201.

Once all the stones are appropriately cleansed and programmed, lie down and take several soothing breaths.

The first stone to be placed is flint; it lies at the earth star chakra and serves the same functions as it did in the previous exercise. Flint is a tether for the soul to return to your current lifetime, and it will awaken past-life memories.

Place your petrified wood or fossil on the heart center. A cross-section of petrified wood is my favorite tool for this layout because the concentric growth rings of the tree record the progress of the wood's growth much like the causal aura composed of bands recording the soul's evolution. The fossil represents the latent memories of concurrent lifetimes and the opportunity to harvest the lessons of other incarnations in order to ensure a new start with much success in the current lifetime. Fossils bridge the living and nonliving planes of reality, and they help us to cross similar thresholds in the past-life journey.

Apophyllite is placed at the third eye. It awakens karmic memories and encourages understanding them at the mental level. Apophyllite helps grant access to the Akashic records, where all of our concurrent lifetimes are documented. Its pyramidal form points us higher, toward a more spiritual context for the mental body's understanding. This enables us to access the spiritual coding underlying any scenario in this life or other lifetimes. Consequently, apophyllite illuminates the blueprint-related information from your past-life journey in order to provide the impetus to amend or update your concurrent lives.

Selenite is placed at the soul star chakra to direct more light and spiritual support into the journey. Selenite initiates contact with the higher self, and it can expand all of our spiritual skills and talents. It paves the way for the past-life regression with an avenue of light, and selenite also calms and comforts any emotional disturbances that may arise.

Place the time link crystals in each hand with the points directed toward the body. Although you may choose to have one of each variety, one pointing to the past and another to the future, it ultimately doesn't matter because time is not actually linear. The time link carries the frequency necessary to facilitate the journey and to better recognize your soul in its other incarnations. Time link crystals also enable you to engage in a conscious dialog with your concurrent selves, as well as to make changes to the timeline in order to alter causal patterns. Because of these capabilities, the time links should be used conscientiously and prudently.

Finally, if using a stone from the list of stones in the aforementioned section "Connecting to Specific Lifetimes," set the chosen stone on the solar plexus. Since the light body is said to maintain its

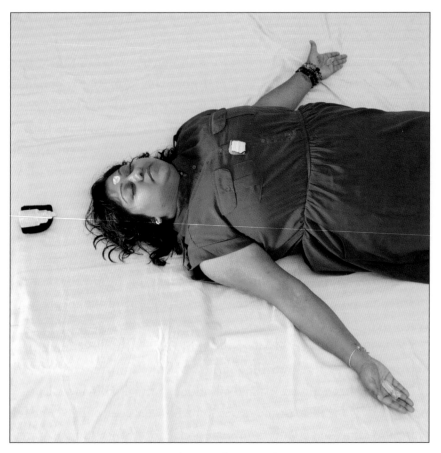

Once the crystals are in place,
continue with your visualization.

connection to the physical body via a silver cord at the solar plexus, placing the guide stone here will serve to direct the light body toward a specific lifetime. For the most effective results, program the guide stone with explicit instructions to carry out this function.

At this point, follow the instructions for the meditation as in the previous exercise. Once you have arrived at the chosen incarnation, take inventory of the scenario in the same way. Thereafter, you may feel free to begin a conversation with your former (or future) self; do so with compassion and respect for your soul's free will. Share how the karma incurred in the other lifetime is impacting you at the soul level today, and help to reframe the decisions that your past (or potentially future) self must make within the context of the big picture.

The crystals that you have placed in the layout will serve to prevent any dangerous changes from being made. Even so, ask that the higher powers take care of any details that must be altered for your soul's highest good. Surrender to this process, and breathe through any discomfort that may arise as shifts arise. When you have finished, thank the higher powers and your previous incarnation. Now you may return the way you came.

When you bring your awareness back to your physical body, be gentle with yourself as you assimilate any changes you have made to your causal makeup. Slowly remove the crystals in reverse order and sit up with caution. You may feel that it is necessary to follow up with cutting any karmic cords remaining from the incarnation to which you have journeyed. Afterward, cleanse all of the crystals involved in your layout.

LEOPARDSKIN JASPER
CAUSAL TUNE-UP

Leopardskin jasper's appearance alludes to its capacity to fine-tune the rhythmic and cyclical functions of our physical and subtle bodies. The spots and circular aggregates of minerals in this rock represent the dials and knobs that symbolically help to reset the regulatory functions governing one's whole being. This can include cycles of metabolism, digestion, or hormonal regulation on the physical level. Additionally, leopardskin jasper can include improving our relationship with time by centering us in the flow of the eternal Now. This helps to maintain a healthy expression of your spiritual blueprint in each moment.

Applying leopardskin jasper in this manner helps to instill a healthy sense of movement in the causal body. It connects each of the chakra vortexes to the causal body, and it allows them to communicate throughout the day. Although it is not especially focused on releasing karmic baggage or negative cords, it does provide a push in the proper direction after these energies have been cleansed through other means. When we carry around a particular karmic pattern for too long it can weigh down the causal body and its functions; using leopardskin jasper can reintegrate the proper sense of ebb and flow in the causal body where the energies may have been stagnant before.

The primary benefit is the ability to seemingly manifest more quickly. Without negative programming or karmic debts piled into your aura, the limitations of previous beliefs and past lives no longer hold you back from evolving and transforming. This also increases your personal magnetism and appears to give you a boost of good luck in all endeavors.

To perform this therapeutic meditation, you will need two cleansed and programmed pieces of leopardskin jasper. Be sure to choose stones with visible circles, rings, or spots in order to emphasize the therapeutic benefits of this gemstone.

Choose a space where you will not be disturbed for the length of the meditation. Sit or lie comfortably while holding one piece of jasper in each hand and focus on the breath. After several moments, move one hand to the crown chakra and one to the base chakra. Hold the stones over these energy centers for approximately two to three minutes. Repeat this process with the stones held over the third eye and sacral chakra simultaneously. Follow by repeating at the throat and the solar plexus. Finally, bring your hands together over the heart chakra and hold both of the stones at your heart for two to three minutes.

Afterward, ground yourself by imagining roots growing from the base of your spine and/or the soles of your feet deep into Mother Earth. Relax as your chakras integrate the energy of the leopardskin jasper. When you feel comfortable, return your awareness to the room and cleanse the stones. It is not advisable to repeat this meditation

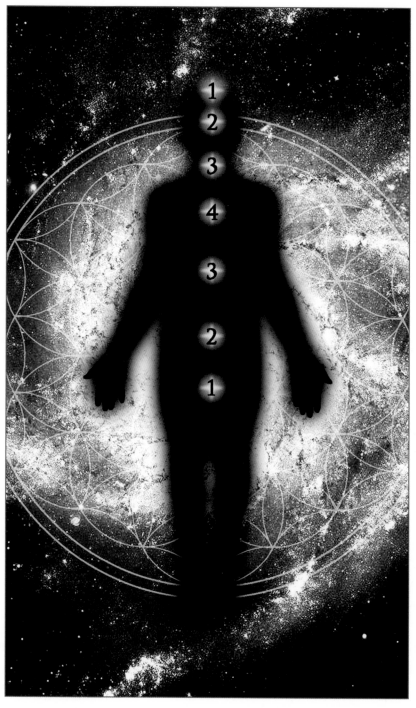

Hold the jasper over the chakras according to this sequence.

more than once a week, as your system will need to integrate the newly established rhythm.

RESOLVING KARMA LAYOUT

Crystal healing generally offers its most profound effects when the stones are applied as a layout, whether on or around the body. The combined effect of the laying-on of stones is much greater than the mere sum of its parts. In this way the law of synergy affords a more powerful and larger energy field created by the crystals chosen. The following layout assists in locating and resolving karma stored in our physical and subtle bodies. You may perform this therapy on yourself on or others; use your sensitivity and intuition to make certain that the recipient is as comfortable as possible.

To create the grid you will need two pieces of petrified wood, one piece of blue kyanite, two pieces of leopardskin jasper, one opal, one piece of obsidian, one piece of rhodochrosite, and one phantom crystal. As always, cleanse your crystals before putting them to work. Program them for resolving your karma, or you can program each of them with the specific intentions outlined below.

Start with the petrified wood below the soles of each foot. It will act as roots, digging deep through your soul's timeline to find opportunities for resolving your karma. Petrified wood will also bring emotional strength and grounding during any release or discomfort that can be stirred up as karma is brought forward in order to be resolved. After it is released, petrified wood will also symbolize your fresh start with a clean slate, and it can engender better appreciation for your healing process.

Rhodochrosite is placed at the solar plexus. Its role is to reinforce freedom and liberation. It sweeps away karma that is lodged in the wrong bodies and returns it to the causal body, where it can better be cleared or resolved. Rhodochrosite can also yield a sweet, gentle innocence; this state of being opens the doorway to resolving

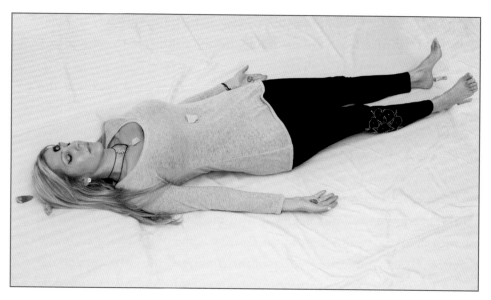

Client with crystal layout

our karma since it reminds us of the grace we know as children.

Opal is placed at the heart center. It elevates consciousness and will help to invite your heart and your mind to be equals in assessing and resolving karmic ties. Your choice of opal will further direct the result of this layout. Precious opals, especially Mexican fire opals, Australian opal, and Welo opal from Ethiopia bring a cleansing fire to the layout. Banded and boulder opals or any opal in its host matrix will facilitate karmic resolution steadily as they pinpoint layers in the causal body one band at a time. Pink opal is especially soothing to the heart center, and it will help soothe any karmic energy that relates to emotional trauma from this lifetime or previous ones.

The next stone to place is obsidian, which should sit on the third eye. A small, polished piece is preferable, and you would benefit most from a black, rainbow, or snowflake variety. Obsidian serves as a mirror of the shadow self, and it can reveal difficult karmic lessons that we have resisted in learning, often repeating our choices that generate more karma. Obsidian is also an initiation stone; since its noncrystalline structure recalls the primordial void of creation, it provides access to the premanifest state, before any karma is accumulated. In this state we are malleable, flexible, and free to release anything that no longer serves.

After obsidian, place the blue kyanite at the causal chakra at the back of the head; it can rest in the space slightly below the skull where there is enough of a gap to comfortably place it. If this is not possible, place it as close as possible while maintaining your comfort above all else. Small, polished pieces work best in this instance because they have no sharp edges and won't take up much space. The blue kyanite will bring this energy center into alignment with the light of the soul. Activating the causal chakra also deepens the understanding of the law of cause and effect, thereby instigating a deep understanding of the "why" behind the karma revealed. When we accept and integrate the lesson represented by any causal pattern, we are better able to let it go and move on.

Phantom quartz is placed above the crown chakra with its apex pointing away from the crown of the skull. This directs karmic energy out and away from the lower centers and out through the inner layers of the aura. The phantoms are symbolic of the old patterns, which we can clearly see and internalize the lessons of without holding on to the old habits or choices that initiated the karma in the first place.

Finally, hold leopardskin jasper in the hands as the crystals integrate their collective energy. This will have a regulating and grounding effect, helping to coordinate the effects of the layout on all of the chakras and each layer of the body. It will also support bringing forward any energy pattern or circumstance that is needed to help in releasing karma overall.

When all of the gemstones are in place, pay close attention to the breathing and allow your mind to be open to any messages or symbols that appear. You may relive old memories or receive flashes of past-life insight representative of the karma being resolved. Whenever the mind wanders, return its attention to the breath and ask for the assistance of the minerals themselves to resolve your karma. After no more than thirty minutes, or for as long it feels comfortable, leave the crystals in place. When the layout has completed its work, remove the stones in the opposite order. Ensure that they are properly cleansed, and bask in the freshness that will ensue in your life.

RELEASING OFF-WORLD KARMA

Some people feel unequipped to navigate life here on Earth and have a persistent sense of longing to return "home." Many possibilities exist for explaining this, including previous lifetimes on other planets or in higher dimensions. Sometimes these people may be newly incarnated human beings who have never experienced a lifetime on planet Earth before. Many such people may be Earthbound angels, ETs, or new souls who are only now learning the joy and pain of embodiment.

Different crystals can help these challenged souls ground and center their awareness more comfortably in the third dimension. Most importantly, crystals and gemstones may initiate a release of the causal attachment to their previous experiences on their soul's journey and help them to develop more resistance to the karmic patterns on Earth. Aquamarine is essential for angelic beings who now feel trapped on the planet; tektites and meteorites are equally helpful for those people who feel their homes are nestled among the stars.

Begin by gathering together the following stones: two pieces of petrified wood, amber, labradorite, shungite, and a stone to represent the karma you wish to resolve. Examples of this latter include

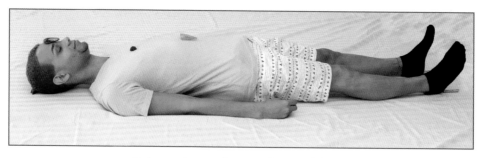

Releasing karma from nonhuman lifetimes

aquamarine, for adjusting from an angelic lifetime; moldavite, tek-
tite, and meteorites, for releasing karma from lifetimes spent on
other planets; and selenite, for lives spent in other planes or dimensions above our physical reality. This healing layout can be adapted
to healing other karmic ties from other nonhuman incarnations, too.
Seashells can heal aquatic lives, moss agate can help connect to the
devic kingdom, and fossilized teeth and bones can be used to release
karma stored from lifetimes spent in the animal kingdom. Feel free
to use your imagination.

Each of the crystals should be adequately cleansed and programmed prior to the layout. Next, begin to place the stones on the
body, starting with the petrified wood below the feet. Follow this with
amber on the solar plexus, your guide stone at the heart, labradorite
on the third eye, and a piece of shungite at the causal chakra. Time
link crystals can be placed in the hands for further amplification, if
desired.

The petrified wood serves to help you stay grounded and nurtured
by the earth during the karmic release. It also helps to refocus the soul
on its current incarnation on this planet, especially after the other crystals have initiated recall and release of off-world or extradimensional
karma. Amber awakens the cellular DNA and the past-life memories
kept there. Together with the wood, it helps to initiate past-life recall,
since they are both fossils. The labradorite opens the inner sight to look
past the appearance of any lifetime. It fosters a deep, spiritual insight,
as well as awakens the light body. Finally, your guide stone, at the heart,
helps to direct and focus the effects of the other crystals on a targeted
lifetime or lifetimes. The shungite works much like a sponge to draw
out the stored karmic information through the causal chakra. In doing
this, it purges the causal level of any residual karmic effects of the lifetime in question.

Leave the crystals in place for no more than twenty minutes.
Remove them and sweep through the aura with some selenite to clean
any karmic debris that has yet to be completely released. Immediately

cleanse the crystals and the space in which this therapy has been performed in order to purify and transmute any of the causal programming that may remain.

VIOLET FLAME CRYSTAL GRID

One of the preeminent healing tools of the Aquarian Age is the violet flame. As discussed on page 55, the violet flame is borne on the seventh ray, and it is available to us through the tireless work of the ascended master Saint Germain. As the pinnacle of spiritual alchemy, the violet flame burns through any base vibration and raises it to a higher level. It can be used successfully to transmute ill health, negative thoughts, interpersonal challenges, and negative karma. It is a versatile tool that can be applied to virtually every situation to effect positive change.

When harnessing the power of the violet flame for transmuting karma, it is possible to create a crystal grid using amethyst to create an everlasting flame, which will blaze through any and all karmic patterns attached to any person, place, event, or idea. To construct the grid you will need a large amethyst for the center, and seven smaller amethysts that will be placed around it evenly. The center stone should be able to stand upright either on its own or on a stand or pillow; a cluster, crystal point, polished sphere or pyramid, or a carved, flame-shaped amethyst are ideal. The smaller amethysts should all be similar in size, and they may be tumbled, polished, or natural. You will also want to use another crystal or wand to activate the grid; this crystal does not have to be amethyst.

As you might expect, begin by cleansing and programming the crystals prior to creating your grid. In addition to your normal cleansing routine, invoke the violet flame and visualize it clearing away any unnecessary energy or information within the amethysts and your crystal wand. Following this, write down your intention to use the violet flame for a specific opportunity or scenario. If possible, you may even

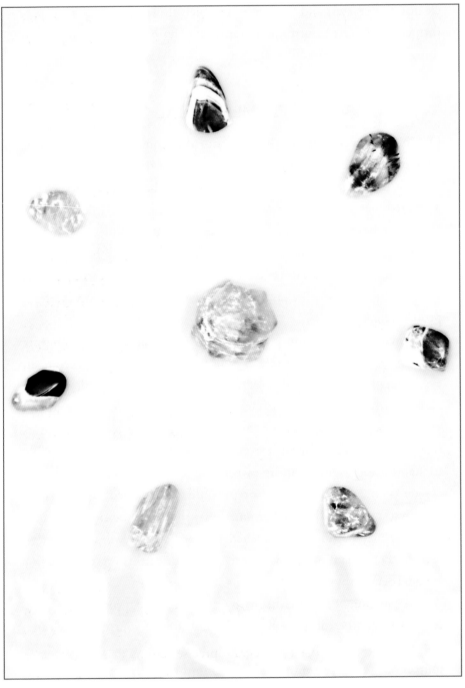

*A configuration of amethyst
serves to invoke the violet flame.*

choose to include a photograph of the subject. Place this in the center of where you will build your grid and put the central amethyst atop it.

Next, build the circle of seven smaller amethysts around the crystal in the center. Start at the top and continue clockwise. If your smaller amethysts are crystal points, aim the points inward, at the crystal in the middle. To activate the grid, hold your crystal wand in your dominant hand and move it in a clockwise spiral, beginning with the amethysts around the perimeter of the grid. As you hold the crystal over these stones, visualize a stream of purple flame beaming from the handheld crystal to each stone in the grid. As you spiral toward the middle, be sure to include the main amethyst in this visualization.

Afterward, and at least once each day thereafter, stand or sit beside your violet flame grid and visualize it sending out a blaze of violet fire to the desired destination. You may choose to repeat an affirmation, prayer, or decree to support and augment this work. When you feel as though the grid has completed its work, change out the written intention for another one and reempower the grid. In this way, you can receive continual support in releasing karma. It is also easy to use this grid for global and familial karma by programming the crystals accordingly. For this, reverse the direction of the smaller crystals so they face outward, thus broadcasting the violet flame around the planet.

REWRITING SOUL CONTRACTS

Healing one's karma can sometimes move along smoothly and easily until a plateau is reached. Oftentimes some patterns persistently resist transmutation and resolution by conventional means; these karmic energies may be part of agreements made in one's soul contracts. When the soul comes into incarnation, certain scenarios or opportunities may be emphasized in order to integrate precise lessons or as a means of remuneration to balance karma's scales. When these contracts no longer serve, it is time to rewrite or eliminate them, and the mineral kingdom provides tools to assist in this process.

Gather the following stones for rewriting your soul's contract: black or rainbow obsidian, chrysotile, apophyllite, an elestial crystal (preferably amethyst), and two pieces of selenite. Ideally, use this crystal layout in association with cutting karmic cords; practice these therapies in sequence in order to remove the cords connecting soul contracts to causal patterns that are currently playing out, followed by this laying on of stones.

After each of the tools has been sufficiently cleansed and programmed, **begin the layout by placing the obsidian on the earth star chakra.** Obsidian anchors and grounds the light body during spiritual healing and soul journeys. Since it lacks a crystalline structure, it also has a strong resonance with the premanifest reality, sometimes referred to as *the void*. Obsidian will act as a guide to the in-between plane in which soul contracts are written.

Chrysotile is next placed at the heart as the guide stone for this healing. Since it is especially attuned to the frequency of the contracts, it acts as a navigator and it will highlight the clauses in our spiritual agreements that are no longer in harmony with our divine life purpose. Chrysotile is generally banded and fibrous; its structure supports sifting through the layers of causal energy surrounding our contracts. In this way, chrysotile can help to remedy some of the karma we have accumulated by disagreeing with or acting contrary to the contracts.

Place a small elestial crystal on the third eye. If possible, use an amethyst elestial; otherwise you may place a small, unobtrusive piece of amethyst just above the elestial crystal. The elestial crystal serves to interpret and alter the geometrical encoding of the causal energy from which the contract is composed. By using amethyst, it also stimulates the third eye and alerts it to any information not in harmony with the spiritual growth and overall nourishment of the soul in manifest form. Elestials purge outmoded data, beliefs, emotions, and behaviors, so this crystal will be pivotal in releasing, as well as transmuting, the limiting aspects of the soul agreements. Since it carries the violet ray, amethyst

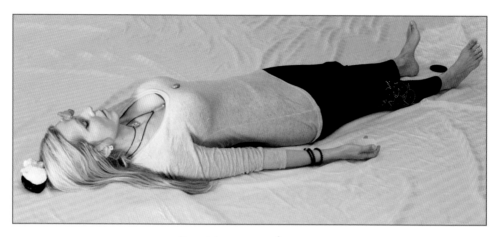

Rewriting your soul contract
with the help of the mineral kingdom

will also invoke the violet flame to transmute the soul's contracts into more supportive agreements.

At the crown center, place apophyllite. It may be necessary to prop it up with a small pillow or scarf. Apophyllite reveals the encoding of the higher aspects of the self, such as the encoding in the layers of the aura and the agreements in the soul contract. Clear apophyllite is almost candescent; it appears as if it is lit from within. This radiant characteristic also helps to illuminate the soul's contracts themselves. It highlights the areas in need of transmutation and helps to realign and reencode them to work in harmony with the original template for the soul. Apophyllite's geometrical makeup is uplifting and expansive, so it can initiate better interpretation of the information held in the spiritual blueprint.

Finally, place selenite in the hands of the recipient. Selenite will promote a healthy flow of energy, especially in its fibrous, striated, or terminated forms. The nature of selenite is practically inseparable from that of light. It appears to exist right at the liminal zone between the material world and the realm of pure spirit. It will usher a cleansing flow to realign the lower self in accordance with the changes being instituted at the soul level. Selenite brings light into the darkest parts of the self, so it will help the most unwilling aspects of one's being lovingly integrate the revised soul contracts.

Leave the crystals in place for no more than fifteen minutes on the first attempt. Short sessions allow you to build tolerance to the types of shifts that occur. Know that it may take several ventures into the contracts to make lasting changes. In this way, you can adjust to the shifting energies more gradually.

If you sense that more "fuel" is needed to transmute the limiting agreements in a contract, Welo opal can be placed at the solar plexus to burn away any and all negative karmic patterns, such as those in the soul contracts.

After completing this layout, each of the crystals should be cleansed.

TRANSFORMING GLOBAL KARMA

As citizens of the planet, we are each responsible for contributing to its well-being and health at the big-picture level. We are invited to help heal and transform our world physically, mentally, emotionally, and spiritually. Within this larger framework, causal healing is a piece of the puzzle to total wellness and wholeness among the inhabitants of our planet, and we can apply our crystalline tools to ameliorate the karmic causes of global upsets.

The initial step toward contributing to the karmic healing of Earth is working on your own karmic debts and patterns. Because the planetary karma includes the sum of all karma of its inhabitants, each time you release or transmute an aspect of your own causal patterns you are furnishing assistance to ameliorating the global karmic imbalances. This is also the easiest way to help heal global karma, as it will not impinge on the free will of any other person. Nonetheless, there are ways to apply the skills and techniques we have learned to enact causal healing on a global scale.

With a crystal grid, it is possible to create a structure composed of spiritual energy that gradually works to increase its sphere of influence. The energy of a crystal grid is exponential rather than additive. Thus it expands outward at a much greater rate than a single-stone application. Crystal grids can be made to commemorate a specific energy or event, or they can be erected for working on a long-term basis. It is important to select crystals and a space to house them accordingly.

My original concept was to create specific templates for a grid to transform global karma. After experimenting in my home and at workshops with students, it became clear to me that grids can be highly personal experiences. Each and every one is unique, like snowflakes, even if they broadcast the same general idea out into the ethers. For this reason I have decided to forego a precise, rigid structure for the "transforming global karma" grid, and instead the following guidelines are offered as suggestions. Chapter 3 offers some simple ideas for crystals that can impact causal healing on a global level. Rather than merely repeating this information, the objective is to look at the most important stones for this purpose and how they impact the effects of the crystal grid.

The central stone of the grid is essentially the generator crystal in your geometrical layout. I prefer to use a large quartz crystal for many crystal grids, which can then be programmed with the exact intention of the entire scope of stones. For this exercise, consider using spirit quartz, which naturally resonates in sympathy with resolving global karma. Large, attractive clusters of spirit quartz will also work to disseminate the healing energy in all directions while simultaneously stimulating a sense of unity and family among residents of the planet. Spheres also make excellent central stones, as they share a state of morphic resonance with planet Earth's shape. Consider a sphere of quartz, amethyst, azurite and malachite, shungite, jade or any of the stones in chapter 4. The choice of stone placed in the center of your grid will color the overall theme of the crystals united around it.

I find that Lemurian seed crystals are also especially tuned to healing our planetary karma. Because they have been seeded with the love,

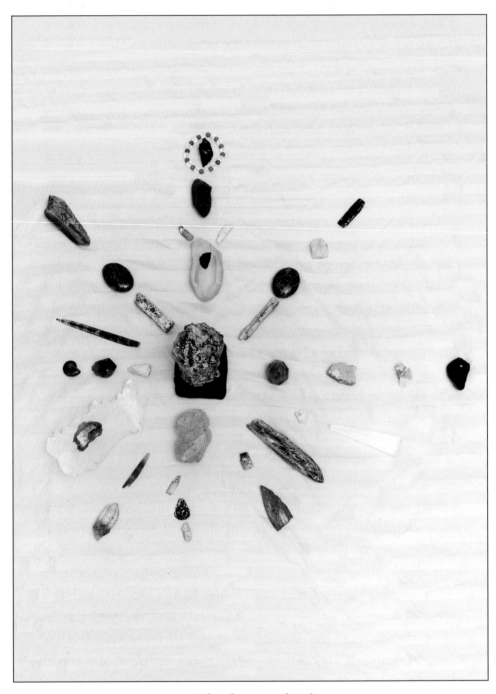

*A free-form crystal grid
for transforming global karma*

unity, and wisdom held sacred by the Lemurian people, they offer balance to the disparate, fearful psyche pervading modern society. Lemurian seed crystals also seek to restore the balance between the feminine and the masculine principles, and they can counteract the karmic cycles begun during and after the Atlantean age. These crystals are now being found in many locations worldwide, so it is possible to create a colorful grid of Lemurian crystals representing many countries around your central stone.

Serpentine serves as a record of Earth's history. Many varieties are rich in tiny inclusions of magnetite, and they will align their mission to the magnetic grid of the planet. The peaceful, relaxing effects of working with serpentine allow for the realization of world peace as the denizens of planet Earth let go of their attachments to differences and seek unity and harmony instead. Chrysotile will highlight causal agreements made for the planet, allowing the energy of the grid to dissolve or transmute any contracts that are outdated and limiting to those who dwell here.

Shungite has an absorbent quality; it will ground the energy of your grid into the planet itself. Since life on our planet is character-ized by organic compounds, shungite's carbon content will also build sympathetic resonance with all who dwell on the planet. It helps to eliminate disruptive energy signatures, including causal cycles, and it can also work as preventive medicine in your crystal grid.

Amethyst and other purple crystals activate the potential of the violet flame for transmuting karma on a global level. The violet flame is the single most effective tool for transforming global energies, and it is amplified when directed through the amethyst. Adding these carri-ers of the purple ray to your grid catalyzes spiritual alchemy, wherein old causal patterns are transmuted into positive energies supportive of spiritual evolution. Placing them into your grid enables it to transmute the karmic patterns being released, such that they will not be able to stick around as karmic pollution.

Additional gemstones can be chosen to support the missions of your causal healing crystals. You can select stones with uplifting, nurturing, and evolutionary frequencies to work as an adjunct with the karmic healing crystals. Allowing your intuition to guide you is a sure method for co-creating a harmonious crystal grid.

With all of your crystals gathered, begin to construct your crystal grid. Choose your central stone, which will serve both to anchor and to project the energy of the grid outward. Next, begin to place the surrounding stones. You may choose to design an elaborate, geometrical grid with precise geometry, or you can simply follow your intuition for a free-form grid. When the last gemstone has been placed, the time has arrived to activate it.

Following the directions from the exercise at the beginning of the chapter, cleanse, program, and activate a terminated crystal. It can be any stone of your choosing, and it should be one with which you have a good rapport. Aim the activated wand at your grid and proceed to trace a clockwise circle around the exterior of the layout. Now use the wand to interconnect each constituent stone in the grid; you may trace the geometries of the grid inward toward the center or just follow your intuition. Generally, I follow this with an inward spiral, which serves to connect each crystal to the focal stone.

Leave your crystal grid in place for as long as you like. If you plan to maintain it long-term, it will be necessary to reempower it following the activation guidelines above. If the grid appears to be diminishing in energy, the crystals may need to be cleansed and reprogrammed in order to restore it to optimal function. In this case feel free to rearrange and reorganize the layout as you feel guided. Your grid for global karmic resolution can be kept in your sacred space, and it makes a powerful focal point for daily prayer, meditation, or other spiritual practice.

TIME LINK PORTAL

The time link crystal is one of the most versatile and efficacious tools for resolving karma from concurrent lives. A crystal grid can be constructed from six of these crystals; three time links to the past and

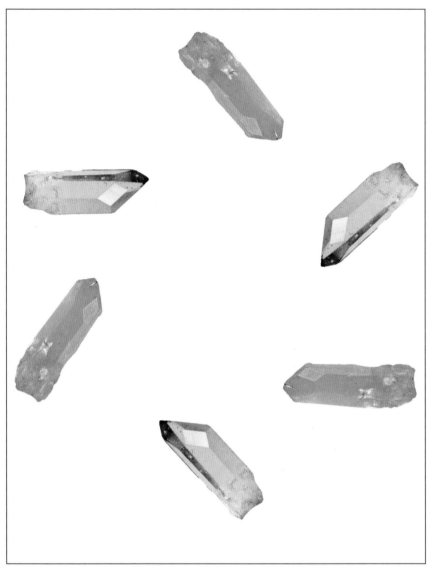

*A hexagonal grid of time link crystals opens a portal suitable
for past-life regression and healing.*

three future time links. This particular grid is a variation on a basic
grid, usually referred to as the Star of David. Unlike the traditional
Star of David configuration, however, the six crystals are not placed
with the terminations pointed toward the center. Instead, follow the

directions in the accompanying illustration, wherein the crystals' points follow the perimeter of each triangle.

Use the time links with windows to the future for the upper triangle, and the lower one will be made from the past time links. The overall formation of this simple grid creates a whirling vortex of energy, rather like a portal or a wormhole. The configuration can be used as a large layout in which you can lie or sit for meditation or other crystal therapies; smaller versions can be used to broadcast a particular energy or intention throughout all timelines. For optimal efficacy, start with crystals that have been cleansed, programmed, and activated. In lieu of a specific intention, try programming these crystals with Marcel Vogel's recommended objective: peace, well-being, and love.

After setting each crystal in its correct position, use another activated crystal, of any type you prefer, to activate the grid. This stage coordinates the efforts of each constituent element of a grid, enabling them to work synergistically. Begin by tracing each triangle, imagining a beam or thread of light being emitted by the crystal in your hand. As you pass it over each stone, visualize the crystals connecting to one another in sequence, with the same thread of light enjoining them. After tracing each triangle separately, continue the activation by tracing a counterclockwise circle along the perimeter of the grid and bring the circle into a counterclockwise spiral until you reach the center.

Meditating in the time link portal facilitates making contact with concurrent lifetimes. This can be applied toward learning from them through observation, and it can be used to rewrite the decisions (and therefore the karma) of these lifetimes. The crystals work together to create a field in which your consciousness is better able to move beyond the constraints of linear time, thereby easing your way into the experiences and memories of past and future aspects of your soul. Larger versions of this grid can be used to support other healing techniques, such as those described above; place the time link portal around the client first, and follow with any other crystal placements desired.

Making a smaller version of this grid allows you to choose a central stone; this crystal's message or mission will then be broadcast backward and forward in time to all aspects of yourself. Try using diamond or a Dow crystal in order to heal at the blueprint level, as they reveal your innate perfection in each incarnation. This can realign and reframe the decisions of each life to be in better accordance with your spiritual blueprint. You may also use a record keeper crystal, which will project its encoded information to your every incarnation. Try gems that cleanse karma, such as amethyst, opal, and wind fossil agate, too. Hourglass selenite can also be applied with a similar function when placed in the same configuration as the time link crystals.

When your work is finished, remove and deactivate the crystals being employed. Do not leave this crystal grid erected full-time. It is important to disassemble it between uses in order to prevent any wayward energies from interfering with time and space. Be respectful of the natural order of the universe and apply this technique with conscious and conscientious objectives only.

BLUEPRINT HEALING LAYOUT

Communing with your spiritual blueprint can be one of the most eye-opening of all healing experiences. When using crystals to facilitate blueprint-level healing, great care must be taken. Because the crystal-line perfection offered by the mineral kingdom is an unfettered manifestation of each stone's own blueprint, these masters of perfection can have tremendous, sometimes unanticipated effects. Ideally, this advanced exercise should be reserved for after you have gained experience through a sufficient amount of meditation and hands-on healing with stones. You may also prepare thoroughly by drinking aquamarine-infused water and meditating with a Dow crystal for one or more weeks before engaging in this healing layout.

In developing this exercise, my initial goal was to co-create a technique that could enable practitioners to rewrite the patterning of their spiritual templates. There is an inherent risk in this, however, because altering vital information at the blueprint level can cause chaos in your life here in the third dimension. Instead, the objective of this crystal layout works from the perspective that our blueprints are innately encoded for perfection and that any friction or disharmony in our lives is a result of causal patterns such as accrued karma, as well as other energy patterns that are inhibiting the full expression of your divinely perfect nature. Thus this layout brings you into better communication with your blueprint in order to make adjustments on all levels of your being.

The stones required for this layout should be cleansed and programmed. I chose to program each type of mineral individually with its specific purpose in the healing grid. If facilitating this layout for another person, then you can build it from the earth star chakra upward. If performing it on yourself it can be challenging to do so in that order, so place the stones at the earth star and soul star chakras before lying down, and place the rest of the crystals in the normal order. You will need to gather the following stones for this exercise: one smoky elestial quartz, two pieces of black jade, one Dow crystal, four pieces of aquamarine, one apophyllite pyramid, blue kyanite, a trigonic quartz, and a white or clear selenite crystal. Two polished or tumbled pieces of leopardskin jasper in the hands will round out the layout.

The elestial crystal is placed at the earth star chakra, with its termination facing downward if it has a main point. Elestials draw the consciousness into the soul patterning beyond the person's incarnation's template. They help us to see what is encoded in the soul that is common to all expressions or lifetimes. They provide a sense of continuity and unity. Elestial quartz also helps to sort through karmic or causal encoding, and it will purge patterns no longer relevant to the soul's mission. Placed at the earth star, the smoky elestial will act as a grounding tool, anchoring your divine life purpose into the Earth plane so that you can express your soul's evolutionary purpose with each and every step you take.

Black jade is placed near the base chakra; set one on each of

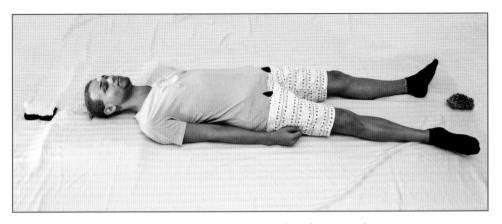

*Place the crystals according to this photo in order
to connect to your spiritual blueprint.*

the groin points, on or near the hip joints. Black jade is grounding, nurturing, and peaceful. Jade itself recalls a sense of timelessness, wherein it invites the consciousness into the awareness of the true self. This spiritual nature exists outside of time, and it is in this same realm that the blueprint is found. Black jade is higher in iron than ordinary green jade, and I chose to use Arizona black jade for its exceptional magnetite content. It serves to draw the higher energies down into physicality, and the magnetite in particular emphasizes re-creating or reattuning the physical body to be a perfect conduit for the blueprint in 3-D. Nephrite jade, in particular, vitalizes the connective tissues because of its structure, therefore it allows blueprint information to be ushered into expression and to become fully integrated by the body itself. It anchors these shifts as the crystals in the upper part of the layout release karma and activate the full potential of the blueprint.

At the heart center, build a grid with a Dow crystal and four pieces of aquamarine. The Dow should be as regular in form as possible; if it contains a phantom it is an even more powerful catalyst for this exercise. Place the Dow point upward and surround it with the four aquamarine crystals as shown. The Dow's perfect geometry engages your being with the perfection inherent in your blueprint; placing it at the heart invites this mastery and perfection into the core of your being. It is the crystalline representation of Christ consciousness, which manifests when the lower self is in perfect alignment with the nature of the spiritual template.

The aquamarine surrounding the crystal at the heart first initiates a phase of releasing any of the causal patterning that has dimmed the expression of your blueprint. The nature of aquamarine is inherently illuminating and cleansing, so it stimulates the act of letting go of any pattern, belief, or behavior that is in conflict with your blueprint. This enables you to be set free of any physical, mental, emotional, spiritual, and karmic limitations that are preventing your spiritual perfection from manifesting in physicality. Aquamarine pushes us into a state of "energetic liquidity." As we become more fluid, we respond better to the information held in the blueprint itself, and we will therefore be more likely to act in accordance with this guide-line of the soul. Traditionally, aquamarine is used as a tool to inspire courage; in this layout it fosters the courage needed to make positive changes in your life so that you can better live and express your innately perfect nature.

Apophyllite is placed at the third eye to facilitate access to the spiritual realms. It encourages astral travel and journeying to the Akashic records and permits better integration of spiritual lessons. In this way apophyllite eases the retrieval of information from the blueprint. By situating a natural pyramid of apophyllite on the third eye, a clarifying effect takes place that fosters a better ability to "read" the patterning of the blueprint and to translate this directive into your life. Since the mind shapes our reality, this seeds the perfection of the blueprint into the mental plane.

Kyanite is placed at the causal chakra. For practical reasons, a smooth or polished piece of kyanite works best, since the back of the skull may be lying against or on top of it. Blue kyanite triggers the causal chakra to respond to the high frequency of light being projected to it by the soul star chakra. Kyanite's message of cause and effect helps to maintain the purity of the blueprint information without interference or contamination from the lower mind. It also activates the cause-and-effect relationship with the blueprint, with karma, with the mind, and ultimately with the life you live. Finally, kyanite fosters connection and alignment. It brings one into energetic and spiritual alignment on all levels with the spiritual realms, including the blueprint. Kyanite opens the doorway to the blueprint and builds a bridge stable enough for this perfection to cross over into our current incarnation.

The trigonic crystal is placed at the crown chakra. I chose to use a glacial etched crystal, specifically the variety called nirvana quartz, in my work with this layout. The triangular etchings are representative of the soul's encodings, and this crystal is a powerful tool for any form of soul journey. According to JaneAnn Dow, where the Dow crystal "pulls you into holographic memory of wholeness, the trigonic takes you out beyond the soul's patterning to the super-conscious Self."[3] In light of this, the trigonic is an oversoul healer; it can adjust your individual blueprint to be congruent with that of the oversoul. The trigonic guides you beyond the experience of limitations and karmic agreements that hamper your divine light from shining. It takes us into oneness with the oversoul and with Creator.

To open and awaken the soul star, a selenite crystal is placed at this point in perfect balance with the elestial at the earth star. Try to use an elestial and selenite that are similar in size. If your selenite has a single termination, point it downward toward the head. Selenite conducts the pure white light of your higher self; it directs soul-level (i.e., blueprint-level) information into the causal and crown chakras for integration and alignment with these codes. Selenite paves the way through alignment to the higher self and by allowing the density of the physical body to become more permeable by the light. In this manner it is a partner with aquamarine, which also fosters better liquidity and receptivity to the light of divinity.

Finally, into the hands are placed pieces of leopardskin jasper. The initial effect of leopardskin jasper is to further ground and

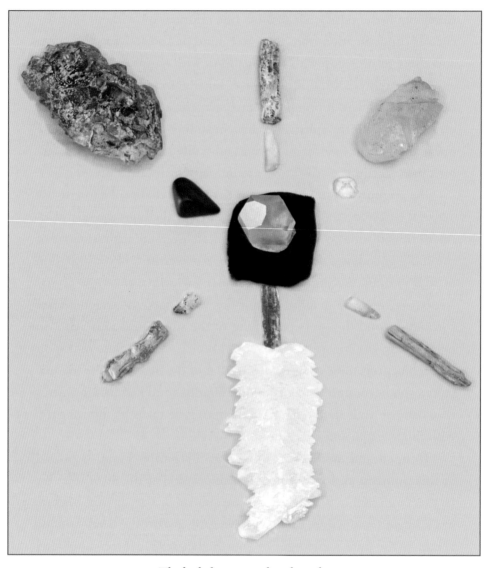

*The body layout can be adapted to
a crystal grid for group meditations.*

coordinate the higher energies flooding the system. It is balancing and stabilizing, and this stone also encourages authenticity. More importantly, it serves to promulgate the benefits of connecting to the blueprint by maintaining the shifts that occur. Isabelle Morton writes that "once old and harmful energy patterns are taken apart or softened, the body may need to readjust its basic processes to assimilate these new patterns. Leopardskin jasper energy can help the body make these adjustments and maintain them. It can also help draw into your life the new things you'll need to maintain these changes."[4] Having one in each hand completes the energetic circuit that courses through your being, stabilizing, adjusting, and fixing the new patterning into place. It helps to reset your presence and timing such that you are better attuned to the rhythmic encoding of the spiritual template.

When all the crystals have been placed, remain calm and relaxed as you focus on the breath. Allow yourself to breathe slowly and comfortably. Pay special attention to any places in your physical body experiencing new or different sensations during the crystal layout. It is important to remain free of judgment or attachment to any outcome. If the mind wanders, bring it back to the breath.

Leave the stones in place for approximately fifteen to twenty minutes; any longer is likely to cause discomfort or dizziness upon return to ordinary, waking consciousness. Leave the leopardskin jasper in place as you remove the rest of the stones in the opposite order in which you placed them. Rest for a few moments, and then perform the aforementioned leopardskin jasper causal tune-up therapy in order to more fully accept and perpetuate the benefits of the exercise. This meditative experience is sometimes disorienting, so take time to ground and center yourself thoroughly once it is complete. Consider following the meditation with a cool glass of aquamarine essence.

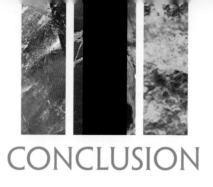

CONCLUSION

EARTH AND ITS INHABITANTS stand at the precipice of a singular and pivotal moment in the course of planetary and personal evolution. For thousands of years, humankind has been undergoing a learning process. We have been recovering from the fall of Atlantis and Lemuria, and our present-day consciousness is finally catching up to that of these legendary civilizations. However, the only way to take the next step forward is to clear the last vestiges of the past in order to make room to really own our collective future.

War, wealth inequality, oppression, and many other forms of social injustice appear to be coming to a head more now than ever. These challenges are the wounds our world wants to close up; we are in the midst of a planetary healing crisis that appears to be worsening just before it gets better. This is the final hurdle before stepping wholeheartedly into the Aquarian Age, where love, unity, integrity, and innovation will draw human consciousness together in love. It is our duty as the spiritually awakened cognoscenti of the world to step up and take responsibility for the karmic patterns limiting our planet from progressing.

Unlike ever before, the spiritual hierarchy has granted special dispensation to the denizens of Earth. We can move forward in our evolutionary path without transmuting every last speck of negative karma. Critical mass has been lowered to a scant majority, where only 51 percent must be cleared in order to shift the entire world. With this one-time reprieve, we can take the reins of planetary healing by clearing away negative karma. The tools available to us through the mineral kingdom enable us to release and transmute karma at an unprecedented rate. What once took many lifetimes over the span of millennia can be accomplished in the here and now. The shift of consciousness affects us all, even people who may not have chosen an overtly spiritual life path. It is now easier than ever to work hand in hand with the higher planes, which enables us to grow and heal like never before.

We are truly in this together. The greatest gift that you can give to the world is to heal yourself. Your karma is all that you are responsible for, and by eliminating your own limiting causal patterns, you free the world from a portion of its collective karma. Now, because of the tools we have available, we can accelerate this process by moving our focus to familial and ancestral karma, as well as the karma of large groups and nations, even that of the entire planet. Humanity has been offered the chance to rewrite soul contracts, transmute negative karma, and help our neighbors in ways never before accomplished.

The mineral kingdom is one of our greatest allies in this process. Since the stones of Earth generate none of their own karma, they lovingly and gracefully offer themselves in meritorious service for the healing and transformation of other beings. The changes in planetary energy have also revealed the most important and timeliest tools for this process. New mineral formations are being discovered each year, and many of these special crystals offer unexpected and dynamic possibilities for healing on all levels of body, mind, and spirit.

By incarnating now, we have elected to participate in Earth's greatest healing opportunity. It is up to us to take responsibility for our own karma, as well as to help transform the collective, global karma. Although it may not belong to any one person, this karma holds us all back, and we can partner with the mineral kingdom, for rocks and minerals are our fellow sentient inhabitants of Earth. Together we really can change the world.

NOTES

CHAPTER 1. UNDERSTANDING KARMA

1. Querido, *Western Approach,* xxii.
2. Ibid., xxii–xxvi.
3. Ginny Katz, *Beyond the Light,* 59.
4. Ibid.
5. Michael Katz, *Aquamarine Water,* 5.
6. Papastavros, *Gnosis,* 152.

CHAPTER 2. THE LORDS OF KARMA

1. www.saintgermainfoundation.org (accessed Nov. 9, 2016).
2. Papastavros, *Gnosis,* 150.
3. Ibid., 151–52.
4. Ibid., 154.
5. Coquet, *Stones,* 188.
6. Ibid., 215.
7. Ibid., 250.
8. Ibid., 264.
9. Ibid., 275.
10. Ibid., 290.
11. Querido, *Western Approach,* lxv.
12. Ibid., lxviii.
13. Coquet, *Stones,* 232.

14. Fairchild, *Crystal Masters,* 23.
15. Virtue and Lukomski, *Crystal Therapy,* 30.

CHAPTER 3. WORKING WITH KARMA

1. Brennan, *Hands of Light,* 53.
2. Papastavros, *Gnosis,* 42.
3. Morton, *Basic Gemstone Therapy,* 161.
4. Raphaell, *Crystalline Transmission,* 35.
5. Ibid., 73.
6. Penczak, *Ascension Magick,* 341.
7. Prophet, *Violet Flame,* 91.
8. Ibid., 10.
9. Cota-Robles, *The Violet Flame,* 42.
10. Nicholas Pearson, "Crystals for Karmic Healing" (workshop notes, Daytona Beach, Fla., September 2015).

CHAPTER 4. DIRECTORY OF CRYSTALS FOR KARMIC HEALING

1. Charman, *Crystals,* 112.
2. Ibid.
3. Michael Katz, *Aquamarine Water,* 5.
4. Melody, *Love,* 193.
5. Simmons and Ahsian, *Book of Stones,* 108.
6. Roeder, *Crystal Co-Creators,* 72.
7. Ibid.
8. Pearson, *Seven Archetypal Stones.*
9. Hall, *Crystal Bible 2,* 121.
10. Ibid.
11. Twintreess and Twintreess, *Stones Alive! 2,* 71–72.
12. Gienger, *Crystal Power,* 278.
13. Bob Geisel, correspondence with author. See also https://magicaldelights .wordpress.com (accessed Nov. 9, 2016).

14. Fairchild, *Crystal Masters,* 23.

15. Cunningham, *Cunningham's Encyclopedia,* 95.

16. Raphaell, *Crystalline Transmission,* 85.

17. Pelikan, *Secrets of Metals,* 48.

18. Melody, *Love,* 312.

19. Morton, *Basic Gemstone Therapy,* 161.

20. Ibid.

21. Pearson, *Seven Archetypal Stones.*

22. Ibid.

23. Raphaell, *Crystalline Transmission,* 73.

24. www.gemformulas.com/healing-necklaces/leopardskin-jasper-peach
    -aventurine (accessed Aug. 5, 2016).

25. Hall, *Crystal Bible: Definitive Guide,* 209.

26. Michael Katz, *Gemstone Energy,* 75.

27. Hall, *Crystal Bible: Definitive Guide,* 211.

28. Hall, *Crystal Bible 3,* 214.

29. Melody, *Love,* 536.

30. Roeder, *Crystal Co-Creators,* 141.

31. Ibid., 142.

32. Lilly and Lilly, *Preseli Bluestone,* 34.

33. Ibid., 76.

34. Ibid.

35. Raphaell, *Crystalline Transmission,* 127.

36. Ibid., 130.

37. Dow, *Crystal Journey,* 247.

38. Ibid., 248.

39. Ibid., 249.

40. Hall, *101 Power Crystals,* 84.

41. Raphaell, *Crystal Healing,* 129.

42. Raphaell, *Crystal Enlightenment,* 65.

43. Ibid., 66.

44. Hall, *101 Power Crystals,* 30.

45. Raphaell, *Crystalline Transmission,* 195.

46. Ibid., 196.

47. Ibid., 198.

48. Ibid., 199.

49. Hall, *101 Power Crystals,* 208.

50. Dow, *Crystal Journey,* 254.

51. Hall, *101 Power Crystals,* 168.

52. Raphaell, *Crystalline Transmission,* 65.

53. Simmons and Ahsian, *Book of Stones,* 356.

54. Ibid.

55. Ibid., 380.

56. www.judyhall.co.uk/miscellaneous/the-top-5-crystals-for-a-karmic-detox (accessed Sept. 12, 2015).

57. Martino, *Shungite,* 67.

58. Michael Katz, *Gemstone Energy,* 241.

59. Hall, *Crystal Bible 2,* 147.

60. Hall, *Crystals to Empower You,* 56.

61. Ibid.

CHAPTER 5. KARMIC TOOL KIT

1. Jensen, *Introduction to Vogel,* 13–15.

2. Roeder, *Crystal Co-Creators,* 53.

3. Dow, *Crystal Journey,* 254.

4. Morton, *Basic Gemstone Therapy,* 162.

BIBLIOGRAPHY

Brennan, Barbara Ann. *Hands of Light: A Guide to Healing through the Human Energy*. New York: Bantam Books, 1988.

Charman, Rachelle. *Crystals: Understand and Connect to the Medicine and Healing of Crystals*. Summer Hill, Australia: Rockpool Publishing, 2013.

Coquet, Michel. *Stones of the Seven Rays: The Science of the Seven Facets of the Soul*. Rochester, Vt.: Destiny Books, 2012.

Cota-Robles, Patricia Diane. *The Violet Flame: God's Gift to Humanity*. Tucson, Ariz.: New Age Study of Humanity's Purpose, 2007.

Cunningham, Scott. *Cunningham's Encyclopedia of Crystal, Gem and Metal Magic*. St. Paul, Minn.: Llewellyn Publications, 1988.

Dow, JaneAnn. *Crystal Journey: Travel Guide for the New Shaman*. Santa Fe, N.Mex.: Journey Books, 1996.

Fairchild, Alana. *Crystal Masters 333: Initiation with the Divine Power of Heaven and Earth*. St. Paul, Minn.: Llewellyn Publications, 2014.

Gienger, Michael. *Crystal Power, Crystal Healing*. Translated by Astrid Mick. London, U.K.: Cassell Illustrated, 2009.

Hall, Judy. *101 Power Crystals: The Ultimate Guide to Magical Crystals, Gems, and Stones for Healing and Transformation*. Beverly, Mass.: Fair Winds Press, 2011.

———. *The Crystal Bible: A Definitive Guide to Crystals*. Cincinnati, Ohio: Walking Stick Press, 2004.

———. *The Crystal Bible 2*. Cincinnati, Ohio: Walking Stick Press, 2009.

———. *The Crystal Bible 3*. Blue Ash, Ohio: Walking Stick Press, 2013.

———. *Crystals to Empower You: Use Crystals and the Law of Attraction to*

Manifest Abundance, Wellbeing and Happiness. Blue Ash, Ohio: Walking Stick Press, 2013.

Jensen, Paul. *Introduction to Vogel Healing Tools.* n.p.: Foundation for the Advancement of Vogel Healing Techniques, 1999.

Katz, Ginny. *Beyond the Light: A Personal Guidebook for Healing, Growth, and Enlightenment.* Gresham, Ore.: Golden Age Publishing, 1991.

Katz, Michael. *Aquamarine Water: Fountain of Youthful Vitality.* Portland, Ore.: Gemisphere, 2002.

———. *Gemstone Energy Medicine: Healing Body, Mind, and Spirit.* Portland, Ore.: Natural Healing Press, 2005.

Lilly, Simon, and Sue Lilly. *Preseli Bluestone: Healing Stones of the Ancestors.* Devon, U.K.: Tree Seer Publications, 2011.

Martino, Regina. *Shungite: Protection, Healing, and Detoxification.* Rochester, Vt.: Healing Arts Press, 2014.

Melody. *Love Is in the Earth: The Crystal and Mineral Encyclopedia—The LIITE Fantastic, and the Last Testament.* Wheat Ridge, Colo.: Earth Love Publishing House, 2008.

Morton, Isabelle. *The Basic Gemstone Therapy Protocol: A Foundation Training Manual.* Manchester, Mass.: The Isabelle Morton Gemstone Therapy Institute, 2012.

Papastavros, Tellis S. *The Gnosis and the Law.* Tucson, Ariz.: New Age Study of Humanity's Purpose, Inc., 1972.

Pearson, Nicholas. *The Seven Archetypal Stones: Their Spiritual Powers and Teachings.* Rochester, Vt.: Inner Traditions, 2016.

Pelikan, Wilhelm. *The Secrets of Metals.* Great Barrington, Mass.: Lindisfarne Books, 1973.

Penczak, Christopher. *Ascension Magick: Ritual, Myth and Healing for the New Aeon.* Woodbury, Minn.: Llewellyn Publications, 2007.

Prophet, Elizabeth Clare. *Violet Flame to Heal Body, Mind, and Soul.* Gardiner, Mont.: Summit University Press, 1997.

Querido, René. *A Western Approach to Reincarnation: Selected Lectures and Writings by Rudolf Steiner.* Hudson, N.Y.: Anthroposophic Press, 1997.

Raphaell, Katrina. *Crystal Enlightenment: The Transforming Properties of Crystals and Healing Stones.* Santa Fe, N.Mex.: Aurora Press, 1985.

———. *Crystal Healing: The Therapeutic Application of Crystals and Stones.* Santa Fe, N.Mex.: Aurora Press, 1987.

———. *The Crystalline Transmission.* Santa Fe, N.Mex.: Aurora Press, 1989.

Roeder, Dorothy. *Crystal Co-Creators.* Sedona, Ariz.: Light Technology Publishing, 1994.

Simmons, Robert, and Naisha Ahsian. *The Book of Stones: Who They Are and What They Teach.* East Montpelier, Vt.: Heaven and Earth Publishing, 2007.

Twintreess, Marilyn, and Tohmas Twintreess. *Stones Alive! 2: Listening More Deeply to the Gifts of the Earth.* Silver City, N.Mex.: AhhMuse, 2005.

Virtue, Doreen, and Judith Lukomski. *Crystal Therapy: How to Heal and Empower Your Life with Crystal Energy.* Carlsbad, Calif.: Hay House, Inc., 2005.

INDEX

Page numbers in *italics* indicate illustrations or photos.

BOOKS OF RELATED INTEREST

The Seven Archetypal Stones
Their Spiritual Powers and Teachings
by Nicholas Pearson

Stone Medicine
A Chinese Medical Guide to Healing with Gems and Minerals
by Leslie J. Franks, LMT

The Metaphysical Book of Gems and Crystals
by Florence Mégemont

Himalayan Salt Crystal Lamps
For Healing, Harmony, and Purification
by Clémence Lefèvre

Healing Stones for the Vital Organs
83 Crystals with Traditional Chinese Medicine
by Michael Gienger and Wolfgang Maier

Shungite
Protection, Healing, and Detoxification
by Regina Martino

Hot Stone and Gem Massage
by Dagmar Fleck and Liane Jochum

Power Crystals
Spiritual and Magical Practices, Crystal Skulls, and Alien Technology
John DeSalvo, Ph.D.

INNER TRADITIONS • BEAR & COMPANY
P.O. Box 388
Rochester, VT 05767
1-800-246-8648
www.InnerTraditions.com

Or contact your local bookseller